HOWARD DEAN'S

PRESCRIPTION FOR

REAL HEALTHCARE REFORM

How We Can Achieve Affordable Medical Care
for Every American and Make Our Jobs Safer

HOWARD DEAN, MD

with IGOR VOLSKY *and* FAIZ SHAKIR

CHELSEA GREEN PUBLISHING COMPANY
WHITE RIVER JUNCTION, VERMONT

Project Manager: Emily Foote
Developmental Editor: Joni Praded
Copy Editor: Laura Jorstad
Proofreader: Nancy Ringer
Indexer: Lee Lawton
Designer: Peter Holm, Sterling Hill Productions

Printed in Canada
First printing June 2009
10 9 8 7 6 5 4 3 2 1   09 10 11 12 13

Our Commitment to Green Publishing
Chelsea Green sees publishing as a tool for cultural change and ecological stewardship. We strive to
align our book manufacturing practices with our editorial mission and to reduce the impact of our
business enterprise in the environment. We print our books and catalogs on chlorine-free recycled
paper, using vegetable-based inks whenever possible. This book may cost slightly more because we
use recycled paper, and we hope you'll agree that it's worth it. Chelsea Green is a member of the
Green Press Initiative (www.greenpressinitiative.org), a nonprofit coalition of publishers, manufacturers, and authors working to protect the world's endangered forests and conserve natural resources.
Howard Dean's Prescription for Real Healthcare Reform was printed on Legacy Natural, a 100 percent
postconsumer recycled paper supplied by Webcom. This paper is acid and chlorine free and is certi-
fied by the Forest Stewardship Council (FSC). The ink used in printing is recyclable and renewable
vegetable-based oil and contains no lead or toxic chemicals.

Library of Congress Cataloging-in-Publication Data
Dean, Howard, 1948-
   Howard Dean's prescription for real healthcare reform : how we can achieve affordable medical
care for every American and make our jobs safer / Howard Dean ; with Igor Volsky, and Faiz Shakir.
      p. ; cm.
   Includes index.
   ISBN 978-1-60358-228-5
   1. Health care reform--United States. I. Volsky, Igor, 1986- II. Shakir, Faiz, 1979- III. Title. IV.
Title: Prescription for real healthcare reform : how we can achieve affordable medical care for every
American and make our jobs safer.
   [DNLM: 1. Health Care Reform--United States. 2. Insurance, Health--United States. WA 540
AA1 D281h 2009]

   RA395.A3D426 2009
   362.1'0425--dc22

                                                2009023345

Chelsea Green Publishing Company
Post Office Box 428
White River Junction, VT 05001
(802) 295-6300
www.chelseagreen.com

		Preserving our environment			
ANCIENT FOREST™ FRIENDLY		Chelsea Green Publishing Co. chose to print the pages of this book on recycled paper and saved these resources[1]:			
345 trees were saved for our forests		energy	water	greenhouse gases	solid waste
		241 million BTUs	125,377 gal.	27,717 lbs	14,620 lbs
		Printed by **Webcom Inc.** on Legacy Hi-Bulk Natural 100% post-consumer waste.			

FSC

Mixed Sources
Product group from well-managed
forests, controlled sources and
recycled wood or fiber
Cert no. SW-COC-002358
www.fsc.org
© 1996 Forest Stewardship Council

[1]Estimates were made using the Environmental Defense Paper Calculator.

HOWARD DEAN'S

PRESCRIPTION FOR

REAL HEALTHCARE REFORM

To the many Americans past and present who have been left behind by our healthcare system. Your time is now.

Contents

Acknowledgments

First, I'd like to thank my coauthors, Igor Volsky and Faiz Shakir, for their long hours, wonderful insights, and dedication to health-care reform.

Many thanks—from all three of us—go to John Podesta, Jennifer Palmieri, and the entire Center for American Progress (CAP) family, who provided much data and policy background. Special thanks to the healthcare, communications, and ThinkProgress teams at CAP, especially Jason Rahlan, Pat Garofalo, Brad Johnson, Ben Furnas, and Judy Feder. Thanks also to Peter Van Vranken and the Herndon Group for supplying helpful information daily. To Jacob Hacker, who was helpful as a policy guru and a sounding board throughout this process. To Nicholas Marshall, Verne Newton, Laura Merner, and Brian Clampitt for their thoughtful review of earlier manuscripts.

Thanks also go to Linda Kingston for her quick transcriptions. To Joni Praded for her patience and hard work in the editing process. To Margo Baldwin of Chelsea Green for her faith and her encouragement in the rough spots. And to Karen Finney, former communications director of the Democratic National Committee, who continues to be an advisor and a friend.

Finally, I'd like to thank my wonderful wife, Dr. Judy Steinberg, who puts up with my multiple projects and long hours, and has been a wonderful resource for this book as a practicing primary care physician.

HOWARD DEAN
June 2009

Preface

In 1971, I graduated from Yale University with a BA in political science. I had no clue what I wanted to do. After washing dishes, pouring concrete, and skiing in Colorado for a winter, I decided it was time to get a real job. I thought it over for a while and decided I didn't want to go back to school and didn't want to teach. Instead, I took the path of least resistance and began a career on Wall Street, where my father, grandfather, and great-grandfather had worked before me. This was during the recession in 1974, and while I quickly discovered I enjoyed learning about money, I wasn't making any. In addition, I realized I simply was not a city boy.

One of my friends, who had also graduated from Yale, had gone back to school to get her credits for all the science courses that would get her into medical school. I admired this enormously and decided to do the same. So I enrolled in night school at Columbia University, took all the chemistry and biology courses I needed for med school, and changed careers at the age of twenty-five.

By this time I was already a confirmed Democrat, having left the Republican Party in college due to Nixon's behavior and his conduct during the Vietnam War. While I was interested in politics, medical school left little time for it. I rooted from the sidelines for Jimmy Carter in 1976 as I struggled with neuro-anatomy and histology. In my third and final year of medical school, however, I found a one-month elective that would allow me to go to Washington. My uncle Bill Felch was a former president of the American Society of Internal Medicine. He got me a desk at the American Medical Association, and I spent a month following Senators Jacob Javits and Ted Kennedy around Washington while they tried to put together a healthcare bill during President

Carter's first term. I had found my calling. I knew then that I would use my career in some way to try to make sure every American had health insurance and adequate access to decent medical care.

While I was in the city, I somehow forgot that I was not enamored with urban life. My three top choices for internship were all urban medical schools! Fortunately, I was rejected at all three and accepted at my fourth choice, which was the University of Vermont ambulatory care program. I moved to Vermont in May 1978 and never left.

In Vermont, a small and wonderful community-oriented state, the vast majority of political positions are part-time. While I was in my second and third years of internship, I became involved in Carter's reelection campaign and got to know many of the state's leading political figures. I was adopted by the old-line ethnic Democrats, who had rebuilt the party to elect, in 1962, Vermont's first Democratic governor since 1853—109 consecutive years of Republican rule. State senator Esther Sorrell, who was Carter's chairman in Vermont, and her sister Peg Hartigan, who ended up being the treasurer for every political campaign I ran until she passed away in 1998, taught me everything I knew about Democratic Party politics in Vermont.

By the time the hard-fought primary campaign between President Carter and Senator Ted Kennedy was nearing its end in 1980, Esther and Peg turned to me and said, "Why don't you run for national delegate?"

I looked at them in shock. "I can't do that. I've only lived in the state for two years. I don't know anybody."

"Well, we do!" they exclaimed together. Esther and Peg gave me a list of 250 people, and their phone numbers, from all over Vermont. They told me to make those 250 calls and to mention their names.

And so it was. At the state convention a month later, I was elected to serve as national delegate. I was about thirty-one at the time, and almost everyone my age was going to the convention for Senator Kennedy. At that point I had not yet married or quit drinking, so during the convention I voted all day with the Carter people and drank all night with the Kennedy people.

When I returned to Vermont, the state chairman, Mark Kaplan, called me into his office. He told me that the chair of the largest county in the state was very ill and was going to have to step aside. They wanted me to run for county chair. I looked at him in astonishment and repeated my refrain: "But, Mark, I've only lived here two years. I don't know anybody."

He looked at me quizzically and with a slightly irritated tone said, "I understand that you don't know anybody, but for some reason you're the only person I can find who can get along with both the Kennedy people and the Carter people, so you'll have to take the job."

And so my political career began.

On August 14, 1991, I was serving my third term as lieutenant governor. I was also still practicing as a physician, and while I was in the middle of a patient's physical the phone rang. It was the governor's office, informing me that Governor Richard Snelling, a moderate Republican, had passed away unexpectedly and that I was now the governor. Over the next few days, I scrambled to put together a leadership team and to reassure a shaken state. On the first Sunday after I took office, I found a moment for myself.

I reflected that this was an opportunity I had never expected, and that it was also an opportunity that I should use to focus on things that really mattered. I later recalled something Jim Hunt, four-term governor of North Carolina, had told me early in my governorship, which seemed in retrospect to encapsulate the moment. "Ninety percent of what we do is urgent," said Governor Hunt. "Ten percent is important."

I wanted to focus my public service on what was important. It didn't take long to figure out that universal health insurance was one of the most important things that I could help bring to America.

From that day in 1991, shortly after I became governor, to this one, I've pushed as hard as I can to change our healthcare system—always supported by an extraordinary staff. As governor, we expanded health insurance with the help of the Clinton administration. One of the highlights of that expansion was that 99 percent of all Vermont citizens under the age of 18 gained access to health insurance coverage. We installed dental clinics in schools serving low-income children, expanded prenatal care, and encouraged the development of community health centers throughout the state.

When I entered the Democratic presidential primaries in 2003, I got into the race for two reasons: first to balance the budget and second to bring universal healthcare to America.

Decades after the subject was first broached by Franklin Roosevelt and then Harry Truman, we are finally in a position in Washington to deliver decent healthcare to every American. Democracy for America—a grassroots democracy organization that grew out of my presidential campaign—is running a Web site called StandwithDrDean.com.

All change grows from the grassroots. Real healthcare reform won't happen without you.

Introduction

In 1988, a thirty-two-year-old woman whom we'll call Claire came to my medical office in Shelburne, Vermont. She was one of the first employees in an early start-up company in Burlington and had had no previous unusual medical problems.

This time, however, she was worried. She felt restless and unusually thirsty much of the time and experienced frequent urination and weight loss. A series of tests ultimately concluded that she had become diabetic. Her disease was severe enough to require daily insulin injections.

She consulted routinely with an endocrinologist, who began the arduous task of teaching Claire all the things a diabetic needs to know. We agreed that I would remain her primary care doctor but that she would continue to see the endocrinologist on a frequent basis initially, and then less so as her condition stabilized.

Fortunately, Claire had less difficulty than most keeping her blood sugar under control, and, with adequate monitoring, good exercise, and terrific teaching from the nurse-practitioners and doctors at the endocrine clinic, she adapted well to her new disease. She was bright, willing to work, and well past the often tumultuous teenage years, which are so difficult for insulin-dependent diabetics.

Four months later, Claire was back in my office in tears, feeling the same restlessness that had first brought her in for a consultation. But this time, the anxiety was not medically induced. I had initially assumed her tears were a delayed reaction to a life-changing illness. Although diabetes can be managed relatively easily, it's nonetheless complicated, especially for someone who for thirty-two years had lived disease-free with the exception of the usual childhood illnesses.

I could not have been more wrong. Claire was in tears because her health insurance company had refused to renew her policy.

The start-up company Claire worked for was unable to afford health insurance, so its employees bought individual policies from a well-known firm in the Midwest. The company claimed that it provided individual health policies at a reasonably low premium, especially for younger people, and promised to provide adequate care, good benefits, and health security. Should something untoward to happen, Claire would be well taken care of. Or so she thought.

The fine print in her contract revealed otherwise.

Letters to the Vermont banking and insurance commissioner revealed that this was a frequent problem, not just with Claire's company, but with many others that worked in the individual insurance market. In fact, this is not a Vermont problem; companies elsewhere have continued to refuse to insure people after they become ill, claiming that the conditions were preexisting, that they resulted from negligence, that the insurance was never meant to cover particular conditions.

While employers are guaranteed the right to purchase health insurance, the great majority of states—which govern the individual insurance marketplace—do not extend the same protections to Americans who buy individual insurance policies. In most states, "insurers can refuse to sell individuals policies based on their health, recreational activities, occupations, credit histories, and a variety of other factors"—and state governments do little to stop them. As a recent Families USA report observed, "[States] are doing very little to provide basic protections for health care consumers and many are turned down from coverage or are charged unaffordable premiums or have their health claims wrongfully denied."

Claire's insurance company earned enormous returns for its chairman and shareholders, becoming successful by insuring only healthy people while rescinding coverage once a person became ill.

I diagnosed Claire in January. By May, her renewal date had come up and she was informed that she would no longer be covered by the company, since she now had a chronic disease. Unfortunately, Claire's story is all too common.

In the March 16, 2009, issue of *Time* magazine, health reporter Karen Tumulty wrote about the heartbreaking and infuriating story of her brother, Patrick, who in middle age suffered from kidney failure. Like Claire, Patrick had a high-deductible health insurance plan that he had purchased in the individual market. "He knew he would have to pay for a checkup himself," so he "always put off going to the doctor until he had to."

Since 2002, Pat had faithfully paid his health insurance premiums, "buying a series of six-month medical policies, one after the other, always hoping he would soon find a job that would include health coverage." Pat's insurer even advertised that its product would "safeguard your financial future" and provide "the peace of mind and health care access you need at a price you can afford." But when the denial claims started coming in, he knew something was wrong.

His insurance company denied coverage for this very expensive illness by claiming it was a preexisting condition. The fine print of the insurance company's policy declared that every six months, Pat would be treated "as a brand-new customer." As a result, anything that went wrong within a few months of his renewal date could be labeled a preexisting condition and excluded from coverage.

More than 14 million Americans receive their health coverage on the individual market, but although these patients pay hefty premiums, only a fraction of the dollars are spent on providing actual care. According to the Congressional Budget Office (CBO), 29 percent of premium dollars in the individual insurance market go toward administrative costs; the average policyholder spends roughly $300 more on administrative costs each year than if he or she purchased coverage through a group policy.

Meanwhile, medical loss ratios, an indicator of how much revenue insurance companies spend on care versus how much they keep as profits, have dropped precipitously in the last decade. That is, as more and more people have become uninsured or discovered that they don't have enough insurance to cover their medical expen]ses, insurers have grown richer. And they employ a series of tactics to protect their bottom lines.

One major insurance company signs up doctors to cover its patients and then reassigns the contract (which is almost always illegal) to a different company, which pays doctors only one- to two-thirds of what the first company agreed to pay. If a substantial number of employers in an area have bought healthcare insurance policies for their employees from this major insurer, then local doctors are essentially held captive by this dishonest practice, lest the health insurer refuse to renew its relationship with the doctors and large numbers of their patients are forced to go elsewhere. In the large group markets run by huge insurance companies that are often publicly owned, the insurers frequently refuse to reimburse patients for things that are clearly covered, counting on the fact that beleaguered insurance commissioners throughout the nation have too much on their plates to chase particular claims.

My wife, who is still a practicing physician, recently recounted to me the story of a man who'd had a physical that was required for his admission into an extended care facility. The insurance company was clearly supposed to pay for the physical, yet each of the nine times the bookkeeper sent in the claim, this insurer made a different excuse for why it wasn't valid. The patient ended up giving up and paying for the physical out of his own pocket—an all-too-common scenario that often applies to more expensive medical procedures as well.

Much has been made of the 47 million Americans who don't have health insurance. But the healthcare reform debate should also focus on the fact that an estimated 25 million working-aged Americans have health insurance but still can't afford to see a doctor. According to the Commonwealth Fund, many go "without needed care, not filling prescriptions, and not following up on recommended tests or treatment." Their stories are heartrending, and it's a scandal that in the wealthiest nation on earth, we cannot adequately cover everybody.

The fact is, there is a huge debate about how much of our health insurance should be in government hands. But our real challenge is dealing with the extraordinary damage that the private health insurance system has done to countless Americans who thought they had health insurance, faithfully paying huge amounts of money into the system over many years, only to find that their insurance company refused to stand behind them when they needed it most.

The real issue in the debate over healthcare reform is not whether or not we should have "socialized medicine." It's whether we should continue with an extraordinarily inefficient system that today features a private insurance industry that takes large amounts of money out of the healthcare system for shareholders, administrators, and executives while denying people the basic coverage that they think they have paid for.

So, the real debate about healthcare reform is not a debate about how large a role government should play. The real issue is: Should we give Americans under the age of sixty-five the same choice we give Americans over sixty-five? Should we give all Americans a choice of opting out of the private health insurance system and benefiting from a public health insurance plan?

Americans ought to be able to decide for themselves: Is private health insurance really health insurance? Or is it simply an extension of the things that have been happening on Wall Street over the past five to ten years, in which private corporations find yet new and ingenious ways of taking money from ordinary citizens without giving them the services they've paid for?

— part one —

PROFILE OF A CRISIS

chapter one

The Trouble with Private Health Insurance

While the individual health insurance market leaves many families without coverage or bankrupt, the great majority of Americans receive fairly comprehensive health coverage from their employer.

In fact, despite the rapidly increasing cost to their employers, they are generally satisfied with these plans. Many, in fact, have been so satisfied that—until now, with millions losing their jobs—they have rarely stopped to consider what might happen to them if they lost the security blanket of employer-based coverage.

Unlike the individual health insurance market, where every person is subject to an underwriting process during which the insurer estimates the possible expenses of providing coverage, employer-based plans spread the costs of insurance across a large pool of workers. Everyone pays the same premium, and nobody can be excluded from coverage because of a preexisting condition. Healthy members subsidize coverage for the sick, and everyone can rely on coverage should they fall ill. But the employer market—where 160 million Americans obtain their health insurance—boasts plenty of problems as well. Since 1998, premiums for employer-sponsored coverage have increased 119 percent. Nearly 9 million workers employed by larger firms (those with 100 or more workers) were uninsured in 2007.

The lagging job market and the economic downturn have had the effect of pushing a growing number of Americans into the ranks of the uninsured. According to a recent report from the Center for American Progress, in March 2009 alone almost 11,000 workers a day lost their health insurance. Nationally, the percentage of Americans "under the age of 65 with employer sponsored insurance declined to less than 63 percent in 2007, from more than 67 percent in 1999," and employers are now reporting that they plan to shift more health costs to their employees.

One recent survey of businesses concluded that "one-fifth of the companies said they planned to add or switch to a high-deductible or 'consumer-directed' health plan with a health savings account, perhaps doubling the percentage of employers who offer such plans." As *The Wall Street Journal*'s Health Blog observed, "A big reason is that employers say the recession isn't just crimping business; it's also expected to drive up their health care costs. Those surveyed said they expect their health benefit costs to spike an average 7.4 percent this year (compared to the 6 percent increase employers originally forecast)."

A Medical Safety Net with Big Holes

The problem is that skyrocketing healthcare costs are increasingly pushing more and more Americans into individual policies, which offer few consumer protections. Individual plans are regulated by the states, only a few of which have taken steps to protect consumers from fraudulent insurer practices. Simply put, the insurance lobby is strong, and many insurers would prefer an unregulated market in which they accept only consumers who are good risks for their business. And as one Families USA report concluded, consumers are left with a patchwork of protections and often find themselves at the mercy of insurers and "the vagaries of states' insurance laws."

Those who are sick have the hardest time finding affordable coverage. Dozens of health conditions—from cancer to diabetes to pregnancy—can render an applicant "uninsurable," and some Americans are unable to buy individual coverage if they have a history of health problems. As Karen Pollitz, research professor at Georgetown's Health Policy Institute, often observes, even minor health conditions, such as hay fever or acne, can trigger a denial by some insurers.

In most states, insurers can refuse to sell individuals policies because of applicants' health, recreational activities, occupation, and even credit history. Only five states prohibit every insurance company from excluding all but the healthiest consumers. One of these, I'm proud to say, is Vermont, which adopted guaranteed issue (meaning no one may be turned down or rejected) in 1991.

Most states pose no limits on how much insurers can increase premiums based on an individual's health status. Many allow private insurers to exclude coverage for preexisting conditions for more than one year and revoke an individual's health insurance policy without advance review by the state.

Healthcare plans in the individual market attract younger, healthier applicants by pairing high deductibles with low premiums. These plans may work for individuals with limited health expenditures, but they don't protect consumers from catastrophic health events. Most applicants are unaware of the limitations until it's too late.

In May 2009, *Consumer Reports* profiled Janice and Gary Clausen of Audubon, Iowa. They reported that they purchased a United Health Care plan through AARP for $500 per month, after Janice lost her accounting job and the family healthcare coverage that came with it. The plan, which advertised itself as "the essential benefits you deserve. Now in one affordable plan," covered up to $50,000 of expenses per year. But when Gary received a diagnosis of colon cancer, his immediate treatment cost more than $200,000. "I didn't think it sounded bad," Janice said of the plan she had purchased. "I knew it would only cover $50,000 a year, but I didn't realize how much everything would cost."

The Clausens are still accruing tremendous medical debt—

debt they will be paying off for the rest of their lives. Their one hope is that Gary, having turned sixty-five, now qualifies for Medicare, a guaranteed public health insurance program, which does not have the shortcomings of the private health-care plan they purchased. If Gary had been five years younger and Medicare not an option for him, they would certainly have lost their house and everything else they own. A real healthcare reform package, which includes a public health insurance option, would give people younger than the Clausens a real safety net. They wouldn't have to wait until they are sixty-five to get decent healthcare coverage.

Incomprehensible Terms, Severe Limitations

In the individual health insurance market, policies often include abstruse clauses and incomprehensible language that makes it very difficult for consumers to figure out what is covered.

Choice is minimal. These policies usually have high deductibles. They also tend to have monthly, yearly, or lifetime caps on coverage. These features do make a consumer's monthly premium lower. But policies with low caps can be particularly problematic: They don't protect consumers against catastrophic loss because of their limited expenditures. For instance, policies with a $100,000 maximum lifetime benefit are common. Many plans—for example, Aetna's Affordable Health Choice (as cited by *Consumer Reports*)—are limited to part-time or hourly workers. *Consumer Reports* cited one plan that covers only $1,000 in hospital costs and $2,000 of outpatient expenses annually. Clearly, any serious illness is not covered by such a plan. The AARP, which is a trusted name for many seniors, makes money from insurance companies by recommending policies to its members. The organization actually does little screening of these policies, and—as in the Clausens' case—people who buy these policies are often left with products that are inappropriate for them.

Consumer Reports also interviewed Jim Stacey of Fayetteville, North Carolina, who bought a policy from Midwest National Life Insurance in Tennessee. "The policy listed benefits including a lifetime maximum payout of up to one million dollars per person." But after Stacey had a bout with prostate cancer, the company paid less than 10 percent of the cost of the treatment.

Stories like this abound.

The Ultimate Hurdle: Profit versus Care

The problem with private health insurance, particularly in the individual market, is not just that it is inadequate; it also stems from companies having to report quarterly profits that must increase every year to satisfy Wall Street. In order to do so, they often have to cut health benefits.

Private, for-profit insurance companies must meet two obligations that are often mutually exclusive:

1. **Their fiduciary responsibility to their shareholders to maximize profits.**
2. **Their responsibility to their customers to give good service.**

Increasingly, the former is maintained at the expense of the latter. No wonder health insurers fear a public health insurance entity run by the government, which doesn't need to show a profit every year and whose efficiency is three times greater than that of the best private competitor.

chapter two

Healthcare Reform Is Business Reform

When I was governor, there was a group of very conservative small business people with whom I'd been at odds politically for some time. In Vermont, everything is personal, so I telephoned the executive director and asked to be invited to a board meeting.

A few weeks later, I arrived to meet with them in a modest conference room. There were about fifteen hardworking people, all of whom had started their own businesses and had worked with their hands most of their lives. They had between 10 and 150 employees in their respective firms.

We had a very blunt discussion about some of our political differences around transportation, one of the issues in which this particular trade association was very interested. Then the discussion turned to healthcare.

We were meeting about a year after I had passed a new healthcare initiative expanding Medicaid eligibility for everyone under eighteen years of age who lived in a family with an income of less than $65,000 (in current dollars) in Vermont. In other words, with the help of a waiver from the Clinton administration, we made Medicaid into a middle-class entitlement for children.

"And what about this socialized medicine program you've put into Vermont for all kids, Governor?" one of the participants asked in a sharp tone. "Isn't Vermont just becoming more and more of a socialist state under your governorship?"

This line of questioning continued, even as I began to explain the program. Out of the corner of my eye I saw the chairman of the association, a beefy, fortyish man with a crew cut, who was looking down at his hands and shifting uncomfortably in his seat. In a flash, I turned to him and asked, "Well, Pat, what do you think about this?" He shot me a surprised glance, but said nothing. Finally, in a low but audible voice, he growled, "Well, Governor, I have to admit, after you passed that program I took all my kids and my employees' kids off my health insurance plan and put them on yours. It saved me quite a bit of money."

There was another long pause before I helpfully chimed in, "See, folks? What you call socialized medicine has made a big difference in money savings for your businesses. This industry is a tough industry with pretty narrow margins. This program just made your margins bigger."

I told them then what I still believe today. A lot of top politicians in both parties talk about doing something for small business. If you want to help small businesses, at least let them pay lower health insurance premiums. In this case, we did so by expanding state-sponsored health insurance for children, allowing employees with children to sign up for individual or spousal plans rather than family plans, thereby saving their employers about 25 percent on each plan.

Restoring the Competitive Edge:
The Fix That Helps Keep American Industry Alive

To fix our economy, we need to begin by fixing our healthcare system. Consider these facts: Over the past several years, for each car produced, General Motors has spent more money on health insurance for the people making the car than on the steel to build it. Starbucks spends more on healthcare than it does on coffee beans. And manufacturing firms in the United States spend almost three times more on healthcare per worker than the foreign average.

More than a third of our healthcare dollars get spent on something other than health, while our companies are falling behind their foreign counterparts.

The truth of the matter is that skyrocketing healthcare costs are threatening America's competitiveness in the global economy. Rising health costs prompt fears that more American businesses will outsource their jobs to nations with nationalized healthcare systems, and a number of foreign companies are citing America's growing healthcare costs as a reason to build their factories elsewhere.

The severity of the situation has united business leaders in support of comprehensive healthcare reform. The business community has finally recognized what universal coverage advocates have long predicted: If healthcare costs continue to accelerate unabated, providing coverage will become a disadvantage and millions of Americans will find themselves without insurance.

Thus, the case for reforming the healthcare system is an argument for restoring America's competitive advantage and protecting the principal source of insurance for most Americans.

About four years ago on a visit to Detroit, I was greeted with blaring headlines in the newspapers: "GM Invests Two Billion Dollars in Windsor," read one. Windsor, Ontario, a few minutes across the bridge from downtown Detroit, is the site of major Canadian car plants. General Motors had made the decision at that time to invest billions in creating new jobs in Canada, in large part because doing so in America would subject the firm to the "private" healthcare system that is bleeding American industry.

In 2007, GM reported spending $4.6 billion on healthcare expenses. Healthcare costs have contributed $1,525 to the price tag of every vehicle leaving the lot. GM's director of healthcare policy snarled that "every second of every day, GM pays for a medical procedure; every two seconds, it pays for a prescription."

GM, like many other large American corporations, has become

what Warren Buffet describes as "a health and benefits company with an auto company attached"—and its foreign competitors have taken notice.

In June 2005, despite what Nobel Prize–winning economist Paul Krugman called "fierce competition among states hoping to attract a new Toyota assembly plant," Toyota chose to forgo the added expense of health benefits by locating its new plant in Ontario, Canada. Krugman observed that Canada's national health insurance system was a "big selling point," saving "auto manufacturers large sums in benefit payments compared with their costs in the United States."

Toyota, which benefits from Japan's universal health system and Canada's single-payer structure, paid $1,400 less per vehicle on healthcare and makes $2,400 more per car than American manufacturers.

In fact, many of America's trading partners—Canada, Japan, Germany, the United Kingdom, and France—have healthcare systems that are financed through some form of shared responsibility, where the government, employers, and individuals all contribute to the healthcare system.

The table on the following page shows how American businesses still contribute the most toward the cost of health benefits.

American businesses are paying more for healthcare, but American workers are receiving less coverage. As Senate Finance Committee chairman Max Baucus explained in a 2008 white paper, this is because the cost of employer-sponsored coverage is rising beyond the means of American businesses—particularly small ones—and workers alike.

Remember, the amount businesses pay to insure their employees has risen 119 percent since 1999. But while employer-based plans still cover the majority of Americans who have health insurance—about 160 million—these rapidly inflating costs threaten to reduce that number dramatically. Baucus noted that the recent "erosion in employer sponsored coverage" has become a serious

Employer Contribution Rates and Hourly Cost of Health Benefits, Selected Top Trading Partners			
Country (rank in total trade with U.S.)	Employer contribution rate* (%)	Hourly pay, manufacturing, 2005** ($U.S.)	Hourly cost of health benefits, manufacturing, 2005 ($U.S.)
United States	11.3 overall		
	13.0 for manufacturing	18.32	2.38
Canada (1)	4.5[a]	19.21	0.86
Japan (4)	3.74	18.06	0.68
Germany (5)	6.65[b]	25.53	1.70
United Kingdom (6)	1.92[c]	20.91	0.40
France (9)	12.8[d]	16.93	2.17
Foreign trade-weighted average	4.9	19.79	0.96

Source: The New America Foundation, "Employer Health Costs in a Global Economy: A Competitive Disadvantage for U.S. Firms." May 2008.

* Employer contribution rates are for 2005 for Canada and for 2006 for all other countries. Many of these countries have minimum and/or maximum earnings thresholds above and/or below which the contribution rate is levied. The overall U.S. employer contribution rate is as of March 2007; the rate for manufacturing is for 2005.

** Hourly pay includes pay for time worked, paid leave, and bonuses.

a Maximum; varies by province.

b Also finances cash sickness and maternity benefits.

c Of the 12.8 percent that employers are required to contribute to social insurance, 15 percent is allocated to the National Health Service.

d Also finances cash sickness, cash maternity, disability, and survivor benefits.

problem. The rate of coverage has fallen every year since 2000, "when 68.3% had employer-sponsored health insurance," according to a 2008 Economic Policy Institute report. By 2008, this rate had fallen 5 percentage points, meaning that some 3 million fewer people under the age of sixty-five had employment-based coverage.

Of course, the automakers and large businesses aren't the only ones unable to afford the rising costs of healthcare benefits. These costs keep small businesses at a particular disadvantage.

Helping Mom, Pop, and Other Small Business Owners

Small business owners and their employees—the engines of our economy—actually account for the largest share of the uninsured population. According to one survey conducted by the Kaiser Family Foundation, 58 percent of all small businesses say they're having a difficult time keeping up with the costs of healthcare.

Indeed, mom-and-pop businesses face the greatest struggle in finding affordable, quality health insurance coverage for their workers. Nationwide, only 42.6 percent of all small businesses offer coverage. According to a 2009 survey by the Main Street Alliance, those that do provide insurance offer lower-quality, porous policies that often exclude dental coverage and have higher deductibles. Generally, small businesses have three major disadvantages when purchasing insurance:

- Because the cost of insurance is shared by a small group of workers, one sick worker could increase premiums for everyone in the group.
- Small businesses don't have economies of scale and encounter higher administrative costs.
- Premiums often vary from business to business and year to year, leaving them unpredictable and very expensive.

In some states, in fact, insurance carriers avoid "bad risk" applicants by excluding applicants with preexisting conditions, "rating practices based on expected health needs," and even charging small businesses "higher rates if they have employees with preexisting conditions."

As a result, the number of businesses with fewer than 200 employees offering insurance fell to 59 percent in 2007, down from 66 percent as recently as 2002. The Main Street Alliance's survey revealed that 62 percent of self-employed respondents and

59 percent of small business respondents don't purchase insurance because "it's too expensive to obtain quality coverage that meets people's needs."

Still, some dismiss the argument that healthcare costs are undermining business profits. Certain economists and some right-wing critics maintain that since both small and large employers can transfer the skyrocketing costs of health insurance coverage to their employees in the form of lower wages, providing health insurance shouldn't—and doesn't—hinder American corporations' ability to compete globally.

While it's true that workers pay for healthcare costs in the long run, "employers face a variety of constraints that may make it difficult for them to fully shift health costs in the short run," the New America Foundation concluded in 2008. Globalization and increased competition in international markets make it impossible for employers to transfer higher healthcare spending, and employers typically respond to increased costs by scaling back coverage, dropping coverage, or increasing cost sharing.

Since 2000, employer-sponsored health coverage has already fallen by 5 percentage points; by 2010, 49 percent of employers say they will reduce their health benefit plan offerings. Forty percent of employers will increase adoption of consumer-driven health plans, and two-thirds of employers will move more costs to employees.

The result is a downward spiral. Underinsured workers often fall into catastrophic medical debt; uninsured employees are forced to either take their chances and live without healthcare insurance or try to find adequate coverage in the unregulated individual market.

What Do Businesses Want?

Fortunately, America's businesses are ready for comprehensive healthcare reform. The consequences of allowing health costs to grow unabated have brought business and union leaders and citizens together to fight for change. Among the strange-bedfellow coalitions are Better Health Care Together (uniting Wal-Mart and the Service Employees International Union), Divided We Fail (Business Roundtable, AARP, and SEIU), the Coalition to Advance Healthcare Reform (a group of businesses led by Safeway CEO Steve Burd), and the Health Coverage Coalition for the Uninsured.

In fact, the Main Street Alliance survey found that a majority of small business owners "believe government should provide a public alternative to private coverage" and "are willing to contribute their fair share toward a system that makes health care work for small businesses."

The National Federation of Independent Business (NFIB) has agreed that "the current growth in healthcare costs is unsustainable for the government and for small businesses alike," and the Business Roundtable—a group of chief executive officers of major U.S. corporations—has identified rising costs as one fact that could "impact job creation, diminish the nation's competitiveness and reduce Americans' ability to save for retirement." In fact, even the U.S. Chamber of Commerce, a group usually aligned with protecting the status quo, recognizes that "spiraling health care costs curb the competitiveness of U.S. businesses and constrain tight family budgets."

Still, the struggling auto industry is perhaps most anxious for reform. Testifying before the House Financial Services Committee in December 2008, then General Motors CEO Rick Wagoner said that his company had spent more than $103 billion over the past fifteen years on pensions and post-retirement healthcare benefits. "Obviously if we had the $103 billion and could use it for other things, it would enable us to be even farther ahead on technology or newer equipment in our plants or whatever."

When Representative Gwen Moore (D-WI) asked, "**Wouldn't this have been a great time for GM to say 'We need a national healthcare program in order to stay viable'?**" Wagoner replied, "Well it undoubtedly would help level the playing field for the industry.

"Our competitors do in most other countries have a significantly greater government role," he conceded.

— chapter three —

Our Responsibility

Healthcare reform is business reform, but it is also a part of individual growth and improvement. America must shift from an illness-based healthcare system to a wellness-based model. We need to build something that makes wellness pay and motivates Americans to take personal responsibility for staying healthy.

Yes, the healthcare system is badly flawed—health insurers, providers, and bureaucrats must change the way they do business. But we also need to look in the mirror. Our healthcare system did not evolve by accident. In many ways our system, like those of other countries, reflects our unique culture and our national psyche.

Like many Americans, I believe that this is the greatest nation on earth. We, as a people, believe that we can accomplish anything we set our minds to. That is how we put the first man on the moon and stood up for democracy in both world wars. It is no accident that so many of the extraordinary inventions of the twentieth and twenty-first centuries occurred in America.

However, America's can-do optimism is also partly responsible for the high costs of our healthcare system. A British physician attending a medical conference about fifteen years ago was reported to have quipped, "You Americans believe that death is an avoidable consequence of any illness."

In many ways that is true. We believe that any disease can be overcome through enough research, testing, and procedures. One way other countries hold down healthcare costs is simply by not performing as many procedures. In Canada, for example, a coronary artery bypass graft (open heart surgery) is done one-third as often on a per-capita basis as it is in the United States. This operation, which costs approximately $60,000, including recovery and hospitalization expenses, does not prolong life according to a Canadian study. It does, however, improve quality of life. In Canada, someone with significant chest pain due to heart disease will likely be treated medically for four to five years before undergoing surgery. In America, this patient is more likely to have surgery immediately and be back on the golf course within six to eight weeks. This is but one reason why our healthcare costs are more than 60 percent higher than Canada's.

Ultimately, rather than creating costly new methods to address late-stage symptoms, we should instead be looking at what we can do to prevent heart disease in the first place. **Real healthcare reform is a necessity. Nothing can be accomplished without it. But changing the American lifestyle will also provide greater savings and better overall health.**

Reforming our lifestyle is a difficult task. Our *It won't happen to me* attitude has benefited America, but it has also been an integral contributor to our banking collapse and to a healthcare system that can no longer be sustained.

As a nation, we have to find a way to think long-term about healthcare. **We must develop a healthcare system that is based on wellness and prevention rather than illness intervention.**

Real change will not occur as long as we pay healthcare practitioners for acute care without incentivizing them to prevent people from getting sick in the first place.

Individuals Need to Do Their Part, Too

So our system needs to change; but we must also play our part as citizens. We need to eat less fat, for instance. We need to be educated about its long-term effects—effects we experience not just as adults, but rather from the moment of birth. In fact, education about fat and sugar intake ought to be part of prenatal care and parenting education on a regular and sustained basis.

As consumers, we also have to get our food industry to think about the long-term damage its practices sometimes do to our health. Loading meat products with hormones and antibiotics may make life more profitable for livestock producers in the short term, but it produces astronomical medical costs when we deal with the consequences—most urgently the rapidly increasing resistance to antibiotics, which prevents us from adequately treating human disease. We need to let our food producers know we want food that doesn't put our health at risk.

There are other, less obvious impacts on our health system that stem from a lack of personal responsibility. Maximum choice ought to be a bedrock of every American's life and culture—but not when choices inflict harm, pain, death, or illness on others. Indeed, I believe we should restrict those choices that inflict harm. People who ride motorcycles without helmets cost me money. A lot of it. People who drive cars without wearing seat belts cost me money. A lot of it. People who drive drunk cost me money. A lot of it. Not only are these behaviors costly, but they also render enormous harm to innocent bystanders.

Choice about using firearms ought to be part of that bedrock; it is, in fact, guaranteed in the Second Amendment to the U.S. Constitution. But irresponsible choice or allowing firearms in the hands of those who are not capable of making good choices is not a guaranteed right and ought to be examined seriously, without ideological intervention from special-interest groups that are blindly committed to principles without thinking about their outcome. We need to start making decisions that stop putting people in harm's way.

There are some glimmers of hope that are spreading on the personal responsibility front. I was recently at a school in western Massachusetts that had banned high-fat, high-sugar products from its vending machines. I expected to get an earful of resentment from the students about it. In fact, I got their assent. Not only did they agree with the decision, but a club had started a garden on the school grounds that supplied part of the fresh vegetables used in the cafeteria. Efforts like this are blossoming across the nation.

We still have a long way to go. Obesity—particularly among low-income groups, but increasing in all age and income groups in America—continues to be a major problem. Diabetes is rising in many parts of the world. Our power sources continue to emit not only chemicals that will lead to global warming in the future, but also those that attack the respiratory health of our children and the elderly today.

Change Begins with Education

The challenge is to maintain our optimism by tempering it with mature recognition of the consequences of our actions over time. This means a new way of thinking about health and behavior that connects what we do today with what will happen to us thirty or forty years from now. It will require extensive educational and cultural shifts. Here we should listen to the conservatives. They are correct to believe that in America, we can't regulate our way to attitude change. Where regulations fail, incentives and education must play a significant role as well. There aren't many American conservatives or liberals who believe that obesity, diabetes, and food safety problems are good things. This is an area where common ground can and should be sought.

The point here is that reforming our healthcare system is only the first step. It is not enough to guarantee all Americans affordable healthcare. It is not enough to squeeze the enormous inefficiencies out of the private insurance sector. If individual Americans want a real change in our health, we also have to take responsibility for the choices we make in our daily lives that can lead to bad health outcomes down the road.

No bill passed in Washington can force us to take respon-sibility for our own lives. But we can change the incentives in our current system so that staying healthy saves us money.

Despite the negative things I've said about private involvement in healthcare, it is worth noting its benefits in one area: Nearly all the wellness initiatives have come from employer-based health insurance programs and employers themselves. Fresh food in company cafeterias, subsidized health club memberships, health education classes, smoking-cessation programs, and reductions in the amount of alcohol served at company parties—all these actions have sent clear signals that corporate America is willing to exercise leadership in the shift from an illness-based system to one centered on wellness.

On the insurance front, many employer-based health insur-ance policies pay the full cost of preventive measures such as colonoscopies and mammograms, while maintaining deductibles for traditional visits to the doctor.

The public sector, such as Medicare, has very slowly started to adopt private-sector innovations by paying for occasional physi-cals, and school boards have begun to push for elimination of unhealthy foods on school grounds. Smoking bans have been widely adopted in the majority of public buildings throughout the United States, even—as North Carolina recently demon-strated—in states with strong tobacco-based industries.

But these are just beginnings, and a massive cultural shift, from the grassroots up, has to take place alongside legislative health-care reform. Only then can we save the kind of money necessary to pay for the kind of healthcare system we want—and deserve.

— part two —

A PRESCRIPTION FOR HEALTHCARE REFORM

chapter four

The Starter Pack: Fundamental Elements of Healthcare Reform

Americans need real healthcare reform, not just insurance reform, and nobody should mistake the two. If we get reform that requires insurance companies to provide coverage to everyone who applies, charge everyone the same premiums, and end their predatory practices, that would be great insurance reform. But that is not healthcare reform.

Real healthcare reform should offer coverage to the employed, the unemployed, the sick, the healthy, the young, the old. Everyone. Health reform should give all Americans the choice between private and public health coverage and break the monopoly that private insurers have on our healthcare system.

Real healthcare reform prohibits insurance companies from rescinding the coverage of cancer patients undergoing chemotherapy. Real healthcare reform protects American families from crushing medical debt, requires insurance companies to spend almost all of our premium dollars on healthcare benefits rather than costly administrative overhead or slick marketing campaigns, and provides us with adequate coverage when we need it most. And it does this always.

Real healthcare reform would give us portable, affordable, and adequate insurance. It would patch our checkered healthcare system by establishing a public plan to complement the private insurance market. It would lower costs by restoring real competition and price transparency to healthcare markets and establish new principles of innovation and health quality.

In short, real healthcare reform, unlike health insurance reform, frees our national healthcare and well-being from the stranglehold of private insurers and gives it back to the American people.

Recall that the purpose of health insurance is to provide coverage when it is needed most. Yet for many Americans, health insurance is either too expensive or simply inadequate. As more and more workers lose their employer-sponsored health insurance coverage, they turn to existing public programs and try—often unsuccessfully—to find coverage in the individual market. Nearly nine out of every ten people seeking such individual coverage can't find an affordable option, and most Americans are too young for Medicare, too old for the State Children's Health Insurance Program (SCHIP), and too rich for Medicaid. In fact, if you're an adult with no dependent children, in forty-three states you can be penniless but still ineligible for Medicaid coverage.

Therefore, any real healthcare reform must include the following principles:

Principle 1: Everybody In, Nobody Out

Everyone should have health insurance. As President Obama has explained, "The only way to eliminate cost-shifting, gross disparities between insurance practices, inefficient medical care, and unnecessary procedures is to have a system that includes everyone."

Principle 2: No More Healthcare Bankruptcies

Americans' financial health must be protected. This means that healthcare coverage ought to be affordable. More than 50 percent of all bankruptcy filings result at least in part from medical expenses; every thirty seconds, someone files for bankruptcy in the aftermath of a serious health problem.

In surveys in Canada, where there has been universal health insurance since 1966, the sense of security is often listed as the highest value of the system. All Canadians know that if something happens to them, they will have health insurance that they can't lose and that will take care of their basic needs. Health insurance reform must make that true in the United States.

Principle 3: Take It to Go

An employer-based healthcare system means that healthcare does not travel with employees if they change jobs. This creates one of the most urgent problems facing ordinary Americans who have insurance: They are locked into their current jobs, particularly if they have a medical condition or if they are older. Essentially they are denied promotion or advancement because they can't afford, for health insurance reasons, to take a better job.

There are two ways to solve this problem, and both should be instituted. The first is to guarantee issue. If you leave your job for a better one or one in a different state, an insurer shouldn't be able to deny you coverage because you are too old or suffer from a preexisting medical condition. The second is to give Americans the choice of either subscribing to a private insurance plan with guaranteed issue or using a public healthcare plan (similar to Medicare) that will cover them no matter where they are in the fifty states and territories. Portability is essential for fairness in our system.

Principle 4: Choose or Lose

Americans should be able to keep what they have if they like it or choose something different.

Principle Five: Improved Care, Quality, and Efficiency

Quality of patient care must be improved. I believe this will be an actual consequence of a more rational system—one in which fewer Americans with insurance can fall through the cracks. It will also be a consequence of a system that reorients its payment priorities so that unnecessary care is no longer profitable. And finally, improved care will be a consequence of a system that has reduced duplication by means of a reasonable and universal technology for electronic medical records, hopefully put together by people who know as much about doctors and healthcare providers as they do about technology and software.

Mandates: Are They Necessary? Are They Practical?

During the 2008 presidential campaign, we heard a lot of discussion about whether Americans should be required to purchase health insurance. Senator Clinton proposed this; Senator Obama disagreed, arguing that the problem was not that people did not want health insurance, but that they couldn't afford it.

Both arguments have merit. The case for requiring all Americans to have health insurance is fairly simply stated.

Insurance is a shared responsibility. That is, we all pay money into a pool for a long period of time in order to have money available should we fall ill.

If some do not buy insurance, either because they can't afford it or because they choose not to, then they are so-called freeloaders. President Obama and Senator Clinton both included all Americans in their insurance reform plans. Senator Clinton believed that everyone should be required to pay something into that insurance pool. She argued that it was unfair to have individuals pay nothing until they got sick, assuming that many would sign up for insurance only once they become ill.

President Obama, on the other hand, was convinced that the vast majority of Americans would not refuse to buy insurance until they became ill. Most, he countered, want to be covered *in case* they get sick; they simply can't afford it.

This is a policy dilemma that I regard as important but not critical to the future of healthcare reform. Both sides are right. Senator Clinton certainly understands the insurance market well, and in an academic sense, she is right about the phenomenon of free riders. A twenty-five-year-old who does not have insurance is simply assuming that nothing of any consequence will happen to him. In reality, if a serious problem requiring high medical expenditures does occur, he will get some sort of treatment anyway—although it will be limited. This means that people who have paid in for their whole lives are helping to give this particular twenty-five-year-old a relatively free ride.

President Obama, however, is correct about those who are older. Older people, particularly those with families, do not go without insurance because they choose to. They forgo coverage because they cannot afford it. Therefore, if we make insurance affordable, responsible Americans will purchase coverage.

While I see both sides of the mandate debate, the reality is that Americans don't like being told what to do. I suggest that rather than mandating coverage, we supply health insurance essentially for free to everybody under thirty years of age, while also ensuring that everybody else can afford to purchase adequate insurance. Young people convinced that nothing bad will ever happen to them would likely choose to buy a Harley-Davidson or an iPhone rather than pay insurance premiums. And let's let them; their age group is incredibly inexpensive to insure.

In Vermont, for instance, we made health insurance available to every child under eighteen and required only a modest premium. We did not mandate coverage, however, and approximately 3 percent of children's families failed to sign up. They remain uninsured. But we successfully expanded coverage without raising taxes, relying in part on a Medicaid waiver from the federal government that picked up about 60 percent of the costs.

The over-thirty population is different. Most of those who are over thirty have entered what we would call responsible adulthood; many have families. If these Americans are unable to either get health insurance through their employers or afford a decent policy in the individual market, they would overwhelmingly welcome a subsidy to assure that their families are taken care of adequately.

Universal health insurance for children isn't enough; clearly the responsible course is to make sure that an illness to one of the adults in the household does not inflict terrible financial hardship on the children. President Obama was right during the campaign: People over thirty will buy health insurance if they can afford it. The vast majority will not need a mandate to force them to do so.

As of this writing, the question of a mandate has not been decided by Congress, nor has the White House addressed the subject.

While the question is of academic interest, I think finding a solution to the mandate problem is a relatively easy compromise and ought not present an obstacle to serious, well-meaning political figures who intend to make sure that universal healthcare actually happens.

— chapter five —

President Obama's Healthcare Plan

When Barack Obama was running for president, he laid out a healthcare plan that may well be the most politically savvy proposal I've seen in the thirty years I've been involved in healthcare policy. It bridges the political divide and still fixes our fractured and increasingly failing healthcare system.

The plan is grounded in one simple principle: If you like the coverage you have, you can keep it. You can continue seeing your doctor and hold on to your existing healthcare plan; you may even receive a subsidy to help you pay for coverage. The pragmatism here is stunning. There is no ideological hook in President Obama's vision. Some single-payer advocates will be and have been disappointed, but the truth is, Obama's healthcare team has learned the bitter lessons of the last sixty years: Most Americans like their healthcare system and they fear that a change in the national health infrastructure could limit their choices.

To insure the 46 million Americans living without health insurance and the more than 25 million Americans who are underinsured, Obama has proposed building on the major existing sources of health coverage—the employer-based system and public insurance programs such as Medicaid and the State Children's Health Insurance Program. Americans will have the choice of staying with their employer-based coverage, enrolling in Medicaid or SCHIP—if eligible—or buying affordable insurance through a new national insurance pool. That new pool, also referred to as an exchange, would offer Americans a menu of private and public health insurance options.

In other words, Americans get to make the choice of what kind of healthcare plan they want for themselves. Obama's plan does not leave the choice up to Congress. It does not leave the choice to insurance companies, employers, governors, or other politicians. You get to choose.

It Works for American Citizens

Insurance companies will be required to cover all Americans regardless of their health status or history and to charge fair and stable premiums. Private insurance companies participating in the pool will have to compete on quality and efficiency with a new public plan and offer comprehensive benefits including preventive, maternity, and mental healthcare. Americans who can't afford coverage will receive new tax credits to help make it more affordable and ensure that families don't spend more than a certain percentage of their income on health insurance premiums.

So if you work for a major corporation, or even a small business with only a handful of employees, you can continue on in the system you have—an employer-based one. You would get what the employer offers for a health insurance plan, you would choose your own deductible in some cases, and you would be mostly free, although less so than fifteen years ago, to choose your own doctor, within the limits of the plan's contract doctors. (This is, of course, becoming a much greater problem: Doctors are now beginning to drop various private insurance plans that simply don't pay enough or that exploit loopholes in their contracts to avoid payment not just to patients but also to providers.)

Obama's proposed insurance regulations are very similar to what we adopted in Vermont in the 1990s. If implemented, no insurance company will be allowed to deny anyone healthcare for a preexisting condition, rescind coverage, or charge sicker people higher premiums. These rules are called guaranteed issue and community rating (that is, the group you join will be rated as a whole, not by factors such as illness or age).

The truth is that insurance does not insure if it is unaffordable or unavailable when we fall ill and really need it. Insurance companies are always wary of these regulations. After we regulated the insurance industry in Vermont, several companies left the state. In fact, we were delighted to see them go. We now have, for the most part, a group of solid citizens selling insurance in Vermont, in both the private for-profit and the nonprofit sectors, as well as one of the highest coverage rates in America.

It Works for Small Business, Too

Under Obama's proposal, small businesses will be eligible for a new Small Business Health Tax Credit—essentially a refund, by way of tax credit, of up to 50 percent on the premiums they pay for their employees' coverage. From an economic point of view, this is one of the major benefits to America.

During the campaign, Obama proposed that small businesses with few employees be exempt from providing coverage to their workers. These employees would instead have the opportunity, with government help, to purchase private health insurance or enroll in the public health insurance option.

This is a significant change that offers real support to America's small enterprises. These businesses create 80 percent of all the new jobs in America. Politicians of both parties are forever making claims that they're going to do all sorts of wonderful things to help small businesses—but it almost never happens, no matter who is in charge. While the Small Business Administration is, for the most part, to be commended for making genuine efforts on small business's behalf, the vast majority of small firms have huge problems with bureaucracy. Large companies can hire staff to make sure they comply with government regulations, but small businesses can't afford that kind of overhead. They are simply too thinly capitalized, and significant numbers of them fail every year. Obama's plan relieves them of this burden.

It also helps them retain employees. It is often the case that when a small business becomes successful, its best employees are tempted to look elsewhere in difficult times for better benefits packages and more security. This is how small business loses talent to larger employers. Again, Obama's plan would mitigate this problem—making it a huge economic plus to America.

This is a reform that would dramatically reduce the costs of struggling small firms, remove significant bureaucratic impediments to growing a small business, and boost the ability of small businesses to create jobs at a time when we desperately need them.

It Raises the Bar on Quality

Under Obama's plan, we will have lower cost with better quality. Obama has frequently argued that without lowering our healthcare costs, "we can't insure everyone under the current system without bankrupting the government or bankrupting businesses or states." To lower America's healthcare costs and build an economically sustainable healthcare system, Obama proposes developing better information about which treatments and procedures work best. Currently, most health research focuses on determining whether a particular medicine or treatment is safe and works. A greater federal investment in clinical effectiveness and cost effectiveness that compares different treatments and medical technologies would enable patients, providers, and payers to make sensible healthcare choices. Obama's plan calls for establishing an independent institute to guide reviews and research on comparative effectiveness to provide "unbiased information to doctors and patients."

Refocusing America's healthcare system on prevention rather than treatment will also contain costs. More than 75 percent of America's healthcare dollars are spent on managing chronic diseases, and Obama will require federally funded health plans to cover preventive services such as cancer screenings and smoking-cessation classes. Employers and local communities are also encouraged to implement workplace wellness programs and community-based preventive interventions. While it is difficult to quantify the possible savings from expanded prevention efforts, experts estimate that simply making sure every child receives all routine vaccinations could reduce direct and indirect healthcare costs by up to $40 billion.

Investments in disease prevention, health promotion, and comparative effectiveness research will improve health outcomes and secure better value for the healthcare dollar; investing in health information technology (HIT) will improve health quality. Obama has promised to invest $50 billion over the next five years "to move the U.S. health care system to broad adoption of standards-based" HIT, "including electronic health records."

Moreover, Obama seeks to improve quality by investing in coordinated care. Health providers will be encouraged to put in place care management programs and implement the medical home model to improve coordination and integration. The payment system will also be reformed. Currently, public and private insurers are paid based on the volume of services provided, rather than the quality or effectiveness of care. Consequently, while some patients receive excellent care, America wastes as much as $700 billion a year on tests and treatments that cannot be shown to improve health. Obama's plan aligns reimbursement with "provision of high quality health care," rewards providers who achieve certain performance thresholds, and incentivizes prescription of only the most effective treatments and medicines.

Choice: The Key Factor

Obama has said, "If you like what you have, you can keep it. This is not a major change for Americans who are happy with what they have." There should be no doubt about what this means for American workers who like their doctors but don't like their insurance companies. They can keep their doctors, they can keep their healthcare plan if they like it, and in fact, some of them will get help paying for that healthcare plan.

Obama's plan looks very much like what members of Congress have for themselves and their families—a fact he stated repeatedly on the campaign trail.

Today a government employee can choose among various plans from a menu of insurance companies. Not all are available in every part of the country, leaving between ten and twenty insurance plans from which individuals may choose in any particular area. If you are a federal employee of the military, you get your care from either the armed services or the Department of Veteran's Affairs, better known as the VA. The irony of conservative politicians who've served in the military yet denounce socialized medicine is that they were the beneficiaries of socialized medicine the entire time that they served. They continue to be the beneficiaries of what they call socialized medicine if they continue to get their care, as they are entitled, through the VA.

This leads us to the most important aspect of healthcare reform: Individual choice must not be merely preserved; it has to be expanded. By extending coverage to all, Obama can achieve efficiency, end cost shifting, and employ a more rational financing mechanism. As I've outlined, Obama's plan offers Americans the choice of staying with their employer-based coverage, enrolling in government programs designed to cover children and the poor, or buying affordable health insurance through a new national health insurance pool. The federal insurance pool will include not just a number of private healthcare plans that the employee, or the individual who does not have employment-based benefits, can choose from, but also a so-called public entity. This public entity, which I hope will be like Medicare, is simply a government-run healthcare plan.

Without this option, I believe that healthcare cannot be reformed, will not be reformed, and should not use up any more of the taxpayers' money.

There are many Americans who will prefer to be in the private sector; that is their right. But there are also many Americans who see what Medicare has done for their parents and grandparents and would like to have a similar choice for themselves. That is also their right. It is a right that should not be abridged by lobbying groups, a private industry that profits from the existing system, or politicians who receive large campaign contributions from that industry. It also is a right that should not be abridged by a political wing so enamored of its own ideology that choice becomes an abstract principle to be applied selectively only in those situations with which they agree.

chapter six

Reform without a Public Health Insurance Option Is Not Real Reform

For the great majority of Americans, staying just one step ahead of mounting medical debt is a constant struggle. Medical crises contribute to approximately half of all home foreclosure filings. According to a recent study published in *The American Journal of Medicine*, 62 percent of all bankruptcy filings in 2007 were partly the result of medical expenses; 78 percent of those who filed for bankruptcy actually had health insurance but found that insurance inadequate to cover their bills.

Even as skyrocketing healthcare costs are bankrupting millions of Americans, however, the earnings of private health insurance firms are rising. In most areas of the country, the insurance market is dominated by one or two large providers. Rather than bargaining for lower rates, large insurer conglomerates are transferring the high prices charged by hospitals to patients and padding their profits. As premiums soared, the profits of the top ten insurance companies grew by approximately 1,000 percent. During the same period, insurers merged more than 400 times, but employee premiums increased nearly eight times faster than average U.S. incomes.

The U.S. healthcare market is broken. Large insurers have little incentive to bargain for lower prices. Smaller insurers do not compete on premiums to gain market share; instead, they follow the pricing of the dominant insurer and compete on risk. As the Urban Institute has pointed out, "Competition in insurance markets is often about getting the lowest risk enrollees as opposed to competing on price and the efficient delivery of care."

Health reform must restore competition into health markets and reorient the business model toward quality of care. To do this, President Obama has proposed a new public healthcare insurance plan that, as I have noted, would look much like Medicare.

Medicare: A Model for a Public Option

President Lyndon Johnson signed the Social Security Act of 1965 and enrolled former President Harry Truman as its first beneficiary. To this day, the program is financed through a payroll tax of 2.9 percent, split evenly between worker and employer. It makes every citizen or permanent legal resident who has been in the country for at least five years and is over the age of sixty-five eligible for Medicare. People under sixty-five who require dialysis or suffer from certain debilitating diseases can also enroll.

Medicare is divided into four parts: hospital insurance (Part A); medical insurance, covering physicians and other services (Part B); managed care plans (Part C); and prescription drug coverage (Part D). Part B costs extra and covers outpatient medication. Part D, which is a drug benefit, is far from comprehensive and requires enrollees to pay large out-of-pocket fees beyond a certain amount.

Medicare is easy to understand. All of your working life, you are taxed 1.45 percent of your income; this amount is matched by your employers. When you turn sixty-five, you become eligible for hospital insurance (Part A). Part B is voluntary, but the overwhelming majority of beneficiaries with Part A are also enrolled in Part B. The program includes limited cost sharing. People who wish to have outpatient coverage pay about $100 a month. People who have incomes greater than $85,000 ($170,000 for married couples) encounter greater costs. Beneficiaries enrolled in Medicare Part B may also elect to enroll in a Medicare Advantage plan (Part C), a stand-alone prescription drug plan (PDP), or a

Medicare Advantage prescription drug plan—programs that are channeled through Medicare but administered by private insurers.

Overall, Medicare provides comprehensive benefits at a reasonably low price. It enjoys high user satisfaction and, given its low administrative overhead, delivers care more efficiently than insurers in the private market.

Still, there are weaknesses in the system. One is that billing criteria and rules are not always clear to physicians. The costs of Medicare are also rapidly increasing. While it is far more efficient than for-profit private health insurance companies, it is a very large program. According to the latest Medicare trustees report, the Medicare trust fund for hospital expenses "will pay out more in benefits than it collects this year and will be insolvent by 2017." The worsening economy is certainly a contributing factor, but the real cause of Medicare insolvency is "the ever-escalating cost of health care."

These problems are not Medicare's alone. In recent years, private health insurance has also begun to under-reimburse physicians, sometimes paying even less than Medicare. The bureaucracy of private insurance companies has increased dramatically. In addition, insurers have resorted to selling contracts to other insurance groups that were not originally physician partners and lowering the reimbursement to physicians when they do so.

In both the private and public systems, we're spending too much money on hospital care because we don't invest enough in preventive care—catching a disease early and preventing the need for hospitalization in the first place. Baby boomers, for instance—who make up 17 percent of non-elderly adults but account for 26 percent of those with at least one chronic illness—have a hard time finding affordable/continuous health coverage and contribute to increasing healthcare costs.

Unless we can reform the whole system—using the public system as a lever to ensure cost controls in the private sector—the continuing financing problems will only worsen.

What Would a New Public Health Insurance Option Look Like?

A healthcare reform initiative that includes a new Medicare-like public option would permit individuals who do not receive coverage through an employer to choose from a menu of private and public coverage options. Enrollees would pay a subsidized premium (should they qualify for a government subsidy) and receive the coverage of their choice. The new public health plan would build on the existing Medicare infrastructure and negotiate with hospitals and doctors for the best healthcare prices. Costs would be set through a process of competitive bidding in which all of the different healthcare plans (public and private) would participate to provide standard benefits.

The new plan would also use its inherent advantages to do what private insurers have only promised: control costs over the long term. Unlike private companies—which typically spend between 20 and 50 percent of healthcare dollars on expenses such as administration, executive salaries, advertising, and shareholder return on equity—Medicare has low administrative overhead and the ability to bargain for volume discounts, as the new public plan would have.

Remember, the private sector's high administrative spending is responsible for a good portion of the excess spending in the healthcare system. According to an analysis by the McKinsey Global Institute, excess spending on health administration and insurance accounted for as much as 21 percent of the estimated total excess spending ($477 billion in 2003). Eighty-five percent of this excess overhead "can be attributed to the highly complex private health insurance system in the United States."

The new public health insurance option could use its ability to negotiate for lower prices and volume purchasing capacity to muscle private insurers into lowering their administrative spending and using more healthcare dollars to provide actual healthcare.

According to a report from the Commonwealth Fund Commission on a High Performance Health System, these kinds of proposals would slow health-spending growth by $3 trillion by 2020, simplify the medical billing process (thus pleasing doctors and patients alike), and allow small businesses to finally enroll their employees into a health insurance program that provides comprehensive health benefits. Estimates also indicate that "premiums for the public plan would be at least 20 percent below those currently available for a comparable benefit package in the private market."

Better Care, Efficiency, Cost Reduction: The Benefits of Going Public

Traditional public health insurance plans such as Medicare have been a source of important payment innovations that private plans have often adopted. A new public healthcare plan could therefore serve as an agent of innovation and quality improvement. Simply having universal healthcare formularies (lists of less expensive drugs that doctors can prescribe) by every insurer, both private and public, could make a difference. This innovation has been talked about for decades, but it has never been realized.

Today's Medicare program, for instance, promotes quality reliable care alongside cost containment. Medicare's refusal to pay medical care providers for "never events"—when a patient suffers a knowable and catastrophic mistake—is something other major insurers are now adopting. Similarly, Medicare's development of its provider-payments systems and its investments in measuring and reporting quality care indicators are being copied by private insurers. A new public plan has the potential to do even more "to drive improvements in the health care system" and set the standard for developing new payment models and investing in preventive care and care coordination.

How Will Private Insurers Compete?

When most conservatives and insurance industry insiders read about increased efficiencies in the public arena, they only see red. Conservatives charge that private insurers could never compete with a new public option on a level playing field. The Heritage Foundation argues that "with the government plan, taxpayers would presumably absorb all of the risks, losses, and liabilities of such an enterprise, while private health plans would absorb their own risks, losses, and liabilities. Consequently, from the beginning, such a competition could not possibly be fair in any meaningful sense." The public plan could use its advantages to outcompete the private insurers and drive them out of business.

As Jacob Hacker, a University of California–Berkeley professor and public plan architect, explains, what the critics of the public option really mean is that "they do not want a new public health insurance plan to have any inherent advantages." That's akin to criticizing Home Depot for outcompeting other home improvement stores by using its market clout to negotiate for better prices.

Stripping a new public plan of "inherent advantages"—like the right to use its market share to bargain with providers or its lower overhead and administrative spending—"is at odds with true competition, which does not require competitors to be equal but that they have an equal chance to succeed if they are equally good at doing what consumers want," Hacker writes.

Hacker explains that giving all healthcare plans the same opportunities to attract new enrollees would require the following:

1. The public plan could not be run by the same authority that governs the new regulated menu of private and public health plans.
2. **All plans should play by the same rules:** charge the same rates to all subscribers (guaranteed community

rating), take everyone who applies (guaranteed issue),
provide objective information (comparative effectiveness
research), offer the same basic package of benefits, hold
adequate reserves, and clearly state their terms.

3. **The public plan cannot dip into general government
reserves** to cover its losses.

4. Plans should be **paid different amounts based on the
risk of their enrollees.** At the end of the year, funds
could be redistributed among the plans to ensure that
those with very sick people are protected.

5. Plans should bid to provide benefits within specific
regions. "Once the premiums were set through competitive bidding, subsidies for low-income enrollees . . . should
be **based on some weighted average of public and private
premiums within the region.**" This way, lower-income
enrollees are not always stuck with the lowest-bid plan.

Of course, if the Medicare-like public option could use its
efficiency to deliver high-quality, cost-effective care, it would
attract more enrollees. After all, this is the crux of why conservatives and the private insurance industry so vigorously object to
a public plan. Their real concern is sacrificing profits to competition. Insurance companies, as we know, have increased their
profits—and their administrative costs—over the last decade
while spending a decreasing percentage of their revenue on their
policyholders' healthcare. Forcing private insurers to shave off
some administrative costs and compete with a public option may
very well reverse that trend.

Their argument essentially amounts to the notion that they
are entitled to be inefficient. I don't believe such a constitutional
entitlement exists, nor do I believe this Congress approves of
entitled inefficiency in the private sector.

More Americans will likely enroll in the new Medicare-like
public option, but the goal isn't to eliminate private insurance.

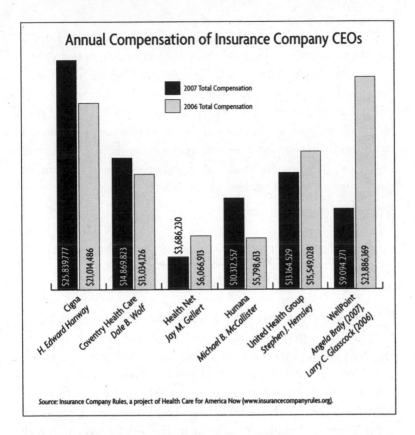

Annual Compensation of Insurance Company CEOs

2007 Total Compensation
2006 Total Compensation

Source: Insurance Company Rules, a project of Health Care for America Now (www.insurancecompanyrules.org).

In fact, private plans would fill an important niche within the new competitive environment.

According to a Lewin Group analysis of Jacob Hacker's public-option-centric healthcare proposal, 28.1 million Americans would find coverage through the exchange in private plans, 65.6 million would enroll in the new public option, and 113.6 million would keep the insurance they receive from their employer. Moreover, in the public plan, "the average premiums would be about 23 percent lower than comparable private insurance for the same set of benefits for the same population." The average enrollee costs in Hacker's public plan would be about $3,250, compared with $4,230 under a private insurance product.

As Hacker explains, "Private insurers certainly will have a great role in providing more integrated coverage options than the public plan would provide." Private plans would also have a "brand advantage" (in the same way that a lot of people would rather have the branded drug than the generic) and "could play an important role" as alternatives that look like the public model but provide "better customer service, nicer marketing and better brochures, but they might also be doing other things in terms of quality improvement or care management that the public plan wasn't."

What Will Policy Makers Choose: Public Plan or Private Monopoly?

Policy makers now have a choice to make: design a system that promotes the general welfare by "providing basic services, protecting the poor and the sick, and ensuring a well-working economy," or protect the monopoly of private insurers and continue redistributing as much income as possible to the wealthy. As economist Dean Baker concludes, "These competing views of government are coming to a head in the debate over national health care reform."

Fortunately, President Obama and 73 percent of voters strongly support a new public health insurance plan. The Congressional Progressive Caucus has even threatened "to vote against any health plan that doesn't include a public plan option." "We have polled CPC members very carefully in recent weeks and a strong majority will only support comprehensive healthcare reform legislation that includes a public plan option on a level playing field with private health insurance plans," explained CPC co-chairs Lynn Woolsey (D-CA) and Raul Grijalva (D-AZ).

But some lawmakers have indicated that a public plan may not be part of the final reform legislation. One senator has recently said that the public plan is just a bargaining chip to "encourage the private health insurance industry to move in the direction it knows it should move toward—namely, health insurance reform, which means eliminating pre-existing conditions, guaranteed issue, modified community rating." **"I think we can accomplish [healthcare reform] without" a public plan, this senator commented in an interview.**

Let's be clear. There can be no real healthcare reform without giving Americans the choice of a public health insurance program. What could be more American than letting Americans choose for themselves, instead of having employers, politicians, bureaucrats, and insurance companies do it for them, as they do so often under the present system?

Moreover, we should not waste $600 billion on reforming the healthcare system and expanding access to care if we can't contain costs in the long term. Without a public healthcare plan, health reform is simply unsustainable.

And there has been no effective cost control of healthcare over the last thirty years. Even though primary care physicians, in particular, have suffered and complained greatly, with more than a little justification, that their working conditions and salaries have dropped significantly under the heels of enormous downward pressure from insurance companies, overall health insurance costs have continued to rise at two to three times the rate of inflation every year for thirty years. In the Medicare plan, while costs are still rising at greater than the rate of inflation, the rate of increase is not nearly as great.

The Lewin Group points out that administrative costs would be significantly lower under a public plan. "First-year national health spending would drop slightly (100 million in 2007—the year projections were done) despite broadening of coverage, new federal spending would be $49.3 billion in 2007. Most of savings come from administrative costs (−25 billion), changes in reimbursement (−7.4 billion), negotiated drug discounts

(–8.8 billion) and more efficient models of delivering care (–11.7 billion)."

While those figures are at some variance with the widely accepted notion that Medicare administrative costs are closer to 4 percent of covered benefits, the difference is still stark. Private insurance costs more than twice as much to administer as does a public insurance plan.

The question that this raises is: Why not require everybody to be in a public insurance plan if it is much cheaper? The answer is simple. You can't take choice away from Americans. This country was founded on the idea that individuals can make their own choices and are free to make their own mistakes.

Furthermore, there will be inefficiency and bureaucracy in any plan, public or private. There will be, inevitably, Americans who are dissatisfied with their plan, whether they've chosen the public or private option. They should be free to change plans. If you have only one plan, no change is possible.

Those who advocate for a pure single payer with no choice for America are most likely correct in terms of the inefficiency of the system, but they don't fully understand the American psyche. Americans want to choose.

Single-payer advocates will not deny Americans choices and in the end legislators won't either—or they will pay an enormous price at the polls, as their constituents are reminded daily that these lawmakers refused to allow citizens to choose and, instead, made their choices for them. If individual Americans are willing to bear the extra costs of private insurance, there is no reason not to let them.

It is incredibly important to understand that the opposite must also be true. If individuals are willing to sign up for a public option, they should be allowed to do so. Votes against the public health insurance plan are simply votes for the health insurance industry. That has not served us well over the last thirty years and it has sought to substitute its own judgments—along with those of its allies in Congress, who have received generous campaign contributions over the years—for the judgments of the American people. There will be a price to be paid for that at election time.

There have been proposals for "public options" that are not really public options. One such proposal calls for copying state plans that feature private insurance companies from which individuals can choose; the bills are split among the state, employers, and employees. The problem with this is that these same for-profit health insurance companies still have to supply a return on investment, large executive salaries, and advertising and administrative costs, all more expensive than in the public sector.

A real public option gives real choices to the American people. A "fake" public option run by insurance companies is not real reform.

— chapter seven —

How to Control Costs

The costs of America's healthcare system are unsustainable. Indeed, because high healthcare costs put many American businesses at a disadvantage compared with their foreign competitors and lead to lower wages and fewer jobs, they are threatening to drive an explosion in the national debt.

Universal healthcare reform will require an upfront investment in coverage and healthcare infrastructure, but to sustain reform we need to figure out a way to lower our healthcare bill. What follows is an examination of how to reduce healthcare spending, eliminate waste in the system, and provide everyone with coverage they can afford at prices that keep track with national inflation.

Reorient the System Toward Wellness and Away from Sickness
This is probably the most cost-effective measure we have for reducing our long-term healthcare costs. Yet in the culture of Washington, where the Congressional Budget Office must crunch the numbers and produce some short-term savings, switching from an illness model to a wellness model will not enter into the calculations. And it's unlikely that Congress will consider this long-term investment when voting on health reform legislation.

But the savings are real. When I was governor, our state Medicaid budget was growing dramatically as more and more seniors needed access to long-term care institutions. In modern America, while our mobility has increased and our standards of living have risen, the nuclear family has not served us well. A generation or two ago it was not unusual to have two or three generations living in the same household. Today this is much less common. When seniors get older and can no longer safely stay alone, their children often transfer them to skilled nursing facilities, because there is no one nearby to care for them.

And while these institutions are an important part of our healthcare system, too many seniors are there for family, not medical, reasons. As a result, they often receive more medical care than necessary, and because many have only modest resources they end up on Medicaid.

Medicaid is generally thought of as a program for poor people, particularly children. But in Vermont, and I suspect in most states, 40 percent of our entire Medicaid budget was used by seniors in skilled nursing facilities.

In the mid-1990s, we received a waiver from the Clinton administration to use Medicaid dollars originally allocated for skilled nursing care to keep seniors in their own homes. Seniors suffering from modest dementia could now be safe and live in a clean environment in their own homes instead of being put in a skilled nursing facility at a huge per-diem cost. In fact, over a period of years, we were able to reduce the number of nursing home beds and reinvest the money we would have otherwise spent on skilled nursing care for seniors.

Expand Access to Coverage

By extending coverage to all, we can achieve efficiencies, end cost shifting, and rationalize financing mechanisms. As Brookings Institute economist Henry Aaron points out, broadly expanding coverage is "a precondition for effective measures to limit overall health care spending." Approximately 75 percent of all healthcare dollars are spent on the 20 percent of Americans who suffer from chronic conditions. To effectively manage chronic disease and invest in real preventive care, we need to ensure that everyone has access to a doctor. As Americans, we're only as healthy as our sickest link. Preventing some of those costly and deadly chronic conditions, including cancer, diabetes, and heart disease, is the only way we can improve the health of the population and lower our astronomical healthcare costs.

Harness the Market Power of Group Purchasing

President Obama's healthcare proposal establishes insurance exchanges that allow small purchasers and individuals to achieve greater negotiating clout with insurance companies. Small purchasers would enjoy greater choice of health plans, greater choice of provider networks, and lower premiums.

Emphasize Prevention

Compared with scientific recommendations, "too few Americans receive preventive services." According to one study, for instance, "only half of recommended clinical preventive services are provided to adults." In 2002, the United States spent $132 billion treating Americans with diabetes, but just $70 billion on the prevention of all diseases. It can be difficult to quantify the possible savings from expanded prevention efforts, but we know, for instance, that if every child receives routine vaccinations, we could reduce direct and indirect healthcare costs by up to $40 billion over time.

Improve Information on Effective Treatments

Today Americans are likely to receive the appropriate care just half of the time, and approximately one-third of individuals seeking care are likely to experience a medical error such as a medication mistake or the wrong lab results. Improving quality could help save lives and contain costs. Estimates of savings go as high as 150,000 lives and $100 billion every year.

Thirty years ago, Dr. Jack Wennberg of Dartmouth demonstrated that in the South a woman was three times more likely to get a hysterectomy for uterine bleeding than in New England, but the procedure did not improve health outcomes. In fact, women fared equally in both areas. This study has been repeated for multiple procedures over the last thirty years and has come to underscore the variation in practice patterns around the country. This is a shocking admission for a field that claims to be entirely scientifically based.

The truth of the matter is, without comparative effectiveness review—that is, research that compares clinical outcomes of alternative therapies used to manage the same condition—we don't know which procedures work, how well they work, and when to use them. As a physician, I don't want insurance company or pharmaceutical representatives telling me how to practice medicine. I *would* like to know whether what I have been taught to do works and how well it works next to other alternatives. Today in medicine the alternatives are numerous; it's impossible for one physician to know everything about a large number of fields, and most of the information we receive about new drugs comes to us in the form of a sales pitch.

The age of direct consumer advertising of drugs isn't making things any easier. Doctors are regularly swamped by patients demanding this or that drug, and the honest truth is that for the majority of patients, many patented drugs don't have a significant advantage over cheaper generic alternatives.

My favorite example is commonly referred to as "the little purple pill"—Nexium. One of the most heavily advertised drugs in the history of America, Nexium is a drug designed to control gastric acid reflux. It costs in excess of $100 for a standard prescription. It has very little additional benefit compared to the generic equivalent, which is available for less than a third of the cost and without a prescription.

Another problem in the drug industry is that when one company creates a huge blockbuster drug, the competition develops a facsimile within the patent laws. Physicians have no way of knowing which drug works better, or whether one of them can produce the same outcome but at a lower price. Comparative effectiveness research informs doctors and helps both patients and medical providers reach better healthcare decisions. It minimizes medical errors and avoids potentially deadly medical consequences. Comparative effectiveness is essential for consumers, and those who oppose it simply don't want you to have that knowledge. They don't want you to know which procedures are better than others. They don't want you to know which drugs are more expensive than others yet yield little additional benefit.

To be sure, comparative effectiveness research cannot be applied too rigidly. A small percentage of patients will respond better to one drug than to another, despite the similar chemistries. For this reason, the decision about which drug to prescribe or which treatment to perform should be made in the confines of the physician's office. Comparative effectiveness research is not designed to stop that. Doctors must have continued flexibility. But making good decisions requires a solid foundation, and if we really want cost control, then we have to give practitioners good information. Conservatives can't have it both ways. They cannot insist they want to control medical costs without giving the information by which those costs can be controlled to those who are making the decisions about how much money to spend.

Comparative effectiveness may reduce the number of procedures doctors perform. But in a country that does three times more coronary artery bypass grafts than Canada (without decreasing the death rate), that is a good thing. The point is, we don't have to have more rationing in America. What we need are sensible and thoughtful choices. We need information.

Greater Use of Information Technology

President Obama has promised to "make sure that every doctor's office and hospital in this country is using cutting edge technology and electronic medical records so that we can cut red tape, prevent medical mistakes, and help save billions of dollars each year." And he's right. Today less than 25 percent of hospitals, and less than 20 percent of doctor's offices, employ health information technology systems. Our fragmented healthcare system and "difficult-to-demonstrate HIT return on investment are just some of the reasons why the market has failed to deliver HIT. For instance, while insurance companies, to a greater extent than providers, could benefit from reduced costs in moving from a paper-based system to electronic health records," the costs of implementation are far higher for providers. According to one study, while providers are footing the bill for HIT, they may experience only 11 percent of the potential gain. Insurance and other payers could reap as much as 89 percent of the gain.

Until gains are distributed a little more equally, medical providers will resist adopting HIT. Fortunately, both Democrats and Republicans have supported the idea of establishing federal standards for electronic medical records and investing federal dollars in sensible medical research.

Very few software vendors bother to visit physicians in their offices to find out how to make electronic medical records work for them. Information technology may save money for insurance companies, hospitals, governments, and even patients, but if they are as user-unfriendly as they have been up to now, doctors and nurses will not and cannot use them. As governor, I saw many vendors who promised us a great deal in technical innovations throughout state government. But in the end, the price tag doubled and the technology took twice as long to implement as predicted. I expect the development and implementation of health information technology to follow this same pattern unless it is implemented with these requirements:

- There must be national standards requiring the technologies to be compatible nationwide.
- The technology must first be tested in small provider settings so it becomes far more user-friendly than it is today.

- Government assistance should be available for small
  and rural doctors' offices to install the new HIT.
  Otherwise, they won't be able to afford it.

The idea is this: Just as the government established standards
for the cell phone industry and then allowed private companies
to build on a single network, setting privacy guidelines for electronic health records would establish a framework for vendors
to develop a system for securely sharing electronic records and
medical data. A Verizon Wireless customer can connect to a
T-Mobile cell phone, and a primary care physician should be able
to transfer medical records and data to a specialist.

Better Management of Chronic Disease

Treating the 90 million Americans with chronic conditions
costs us about $1.2 trillion a year, or approximately two-thirds
of national healthcare spending. Better care for individuals
with these conditions can translate into substantial savings. If
every diabetes patient received the appropriate primary care, for
instance, national healthcare spending would fall by $2.5 billion.

In May 2009, a group of doctors, hospitals, drug makers, and
insurance companies voluntarily came together to present
President Obama with a letter promising to reduce the growth
rate in annual health spending by 1.5 percentage points a year
over the next ten years, lowering overall healthcare spending by
$2 trillion (this represents a 20 percent reduction in projected
growth).

Administration officials estimate that with such reductions, a
family of four would save $2,500; by 2019, national health expen-
ditures would decrease by 3 percent of GDP, or $700 billion. The
fiscal gap would shrink by 5 percent of GDP, and the nation
would inch toward a sustainable fiscal trajectory, according to
projections.

The numbers are significant, impressive, but short on specifics on how industry will reduce costs. Early reports indicate that the group—which is made up of the Advanced Medical Technology Association (AdvaMed), America's Health Insurance Plans (AHIP), the American Hospital Association (AHA), the American Medical Association (AMA), and Pharmaceutical Research and Manufacturers of America (PhRMA), among others—hopes to contain costs by implementing "aggressive efforts to prevent obesity, coordinate care, manage chronic illnesses and curtail unnecessary tests and procedures; by standardizing insurance claim forms; and by increasing the use of information technology, like electronic medical records."

The letter blunts conservative critics who argue that health reform is unsustainable or too expensive and suggests that this time around, industry groups may be stepping up and committing themselves to supporting commonsense—even progressive—cost-containment measures. This is a major political victory for the administration, one it can use to pressure the stakeholders to adopt reforms. Still, as Paul Krugman argues, "the point is that there's every reason to be cynical about these players' motives. Remember that what the rest of us call health care costs, they call income."

— chapter eight —

How to Pay for All This

One of the hallmarks of President Obama's presidency and of his campaign is that, like Bill Clinton before him, Obama understands how all things are connected. The Republicans have leveled criticism that Obama is trying to do too much, too fast. The real explanation for Obama's far-reaching stimulus package, which spent money on healthcare and education, as well as job creation, is simply that Obama "gets" that fixing the banking crisis, while urgent, is also short-term. What he ultimately wants to do is take structural problems out of the American economy. These structural problems have created the excesses we've seen in the finance sector of the economy over the last ten to fifteen years. They include the creation of instruments that no one understands, selling and reselling things like credit default swaps, which initially were intended to lay off risk but ultimately became little more than an option to buy chips at the roulette table, as they were bought and sold multiple times by people who had no interest in the underlying securities or companies.

I believe, unlike some progressive Democrats, that Obama and his team are successfully managing the economic crisis. We have seen some abuses in the Troubled Asset Relief Program (TARP), but that is to be expected when larger amounts of money are funneled into financial institutions that have essentially failed without changing the leadership that led to the failure. There has clearly been some abuse in the stimulus package, which is also to be expected when large amounts of money must be spent urgently to shore up the economy.

Despite right-wing criticism, however, the economic fall seems to have been at least mitigated by these activities. Still, the most fascinating aspect of the stimulus package is what the mainstream media is ignoring: the long-term implications of the spending.

Fixing the economy comes in three phases. First we must address the immediate crisis. Stabilizing the balance sheets of the banks by removing toxic assets will restore liquidity to the banking community. That's what the federal government and its private partners are aiming to do by offering to buy their toxic assets. That will ultimately restore liquidity and allow banks to roll over credit from credit-worthy small businesses.

Next, we must tackle the healthcare system. I have already outlined the damage that our healthcare system has done to our economy. It has made us uncompetitive with our industrial and democratic economic rivals. It is extraordinarily inefficient and delivers care to just 85 percent of the population. In short, the system has not only failed to deliver adequate healthcare to all Americans but also cost hundreds of thousands, if not millions, of jobs because it is simply cheaper to do business elsewhere.

The third fix is education. There was a great deal of money in the stimulus bill for education because President Obama knows that we cannot have a postindustrial economy that succeeds without a much higher level of universal education than we have in America today. The twenty-year plan that is laid out in the stimulus package is not just a short-term fix for the immediate crisis in the financial industry, or even a patch for the intermediate-term crisis caused by healthcare. This fix also involves improving education so that America can flourish again with a knowledge-based economy and replace the jobs that have escaped to our low-wage competitors. For all the talk of retraining that's gone on over the last fifteen years in America, the fact is that without great schools retraining will not happen in our society to the degree it must.

So let's focus on stage two of the economic recovery, which

is healthcare. A universal healthcare system costs money. The Massachusetts Institute of Technology has estimated that Obama's healthcare plan will cost approximately $1.5 trillion over a ten-year period. This figure has been widely accepted, even by Obama's critics.

Most of this money is already in the healthcare system. What the president is proposing is a more rational way to take that same amount of money, from the same sources, and spend that money in a more efficient way by having a more integrated system. It is true that some new money will be required to help people who have no insurance or have lost their insurance. While the care they get is grossly inefficient and very expensive (visiting emergency rooms for strep throat and the like), they would still use more services, although they would be much better services, leading to better outcomes in the universal system. However, much of the $1.5 trillion is simply the federal government absorbing the costs from the balance sheets of the private sector, particularly small businesses.

This is a net gain for industry, particularly small business, because it takes off their balance sheets a cost that regularly rises at 200 or 300 percent of inflation. This is unsustainable in a competitive world.

Nonetheless, the federal government must generate $1.5 trillion of government money over a decade to relieve the private sector of a portion of its burden and to make sure this system works for everyone. This is a staggering sum, even though most of the money is in the system in the private sector today. The president proposed a $634 billion down payment on this sum in his first budget. But that is not sustainable revenue. It is borrowed from taxpayers and other countries, particularly, and most notoriously, China. That revenue stream will not last permanently.

Creating a New, Sustainable Revenue Stream

I propose a revenue stream that will connect the president's solution to global warming with revenues for healthcare.

There are a variety of proposals before Congress to dramatically reduce the output of carbon dioxide and use economic incentives to encourage industry and consumers to produce less of it. We can both reduce our use of fossil fuels and fund healthcare reform. To do this, we'll need to pair a carbon tax with a tax on gasoline.

A carbon tax has been proposed by Representative John Larson (D-CT). That proposal would tax carbon dioxide emissions at $15 a ton and then increase by 10 percent every year. The tax would incentivize lower carbon dioxide emissions and begin to generate $126 billion a year. That amount would grow to $1 trillion every year by 2050.

The federal carbon tax, in addition to a 10-cents-per-gallon tax on gasoline, would bring in approximately $55 billion per year in revenue.

A combination of these two approaches would dramatically reduce our carbon footprint and provide enough money for the president's health insurance plan. Not only does it fully finance healthcare without acquiring any more debt, but it also improves the planet by reducing dangerous greenhouse gases, induces healthier lifestyle changes, and reorients the healthcare system toward a wellness model.

Conservatives and right-wing ideologists will likely characterize the proposal as a "liberal tax-and-spend philosophy!"

To this I respond with the following. First, a tax-and-spend policy is always better than a borrow-and-spend policy, which is what right-wing conservatives have practiced for the last eight years. Second, I think most Americans would be delighted to pay an extra 5 percent on their gasoline bills to ensure health insurance that never could be taken away, even if they lost their jobs. Third, I believe that most small businesses would be delighted to pay an extra 10 cents a gallon on their gasoline bills if they were relieved of the burden of providing health insurance to their employees. Fourth, the very people who would be hurt the most by the increase in the gas tax—working poor Americans in rural states who have to drive as much as fifty miles each way to a job—would also benefit the most from having guaranteed health insurance.

Is this redistribution of wealth? To some extent it is. But so is all of tax policy. The increases in my gas taxes will help the millions of working Americans who are not as fortunate as I am to have health insurance. Better yet, the increase in my gas tax will help give working people the peace of mind of knowing that if they do lose their job or fall ill, they will be able to take care of their children and themselves.

In rural states like mine, the less money you make, the more likely you are to commute long distances for work. Housing costs are simply too high for modest-income people to live near the best job markets. Under the kind of tax I propose, a Vermonter who commutes a hundred miles a day to work would pay an additional 40 cents a day or $125 a year for his or her commute. I know of no American family who would not exchange that tax for afford-able, portable health insurance coverage. These are exactly the people in Vermont who are most likely forgoing health insurance because they can't afford it. So while these hardworking families might pay extra because of their commute, many of them will be getting their first opportunity to afford decent health insurance. They will also have an incentive to drive more carefully, carpool, and use more fuel-efficient vehicles.

This is the classic win-win that is so often talked about in public policy, but so rarely achieved.

Can a Carbon Tax and Cap-and-Trade Coexist?

There are some who believe that a carbon tax is antithetical to a cap-and-trade system. But the global warming challenge, just like the healthcare challenge, is complex enough to need multifaceted policy solutions, not just a single silver bullet.

The truth is, a market-based cap on total carbon emissions and a carbon tax complement each other. We can incentivize the American people and American industry to minimize their carbon footprint through tax policy and rely on the free market to allocate scarce resources. Cap-and-trade would create a market for allocating carbon-production credits in order to meet global pollution-reduction targets. A carbon tax would ensure increased and predictable costs on carbon pollution.

Combined, the two approaches provide economic incentives to transition to a greener economy, ensure our environmental targets are met, and generate revenues to fix the broken healthcare system.

— part three —

WHO'S BEEN STANDING IN THE WAY?

chapter nine

Why Is This So Hard to Pass?

At times, the organized opposition to the principles of health care reform seems overwhelming—the insurance industry, big business, the list goes on. There are too many groups with too much at stake to allow for real healthcare reform.

Reorienting the system from one that treats sickness to one that promotes and nurtures wellness will require holding special interests—whether they be insurance and pharmaceutical companies or politicians—to account.

There have been several major attempts since Harry Truman's presidency to put healthcare reform into effect, with a significant enough government role so the reform is fair and healthcare dollars are spent efficiently and yield comprehensive care for every American citizen. Those efforts have always been framed in terms of what we ought to do for the 16 to 18 percent of Americans who have no insurance. **But while most Americans have an altruistic streak, they are not willing to put a stranger's welfare over their own family's.** Although 16 percent of the American people adds up to a little less than 50 million souls, that is a relatively small minority.

Furthermore, our healthcare system and Congress have something in common. Most Americans do not like Congress, but they do like their own representative. That is why most members of Congress are reelected time after time—even during periods of political upheaval. Likewise, most Americans recognize the significant deficiencies in our healthcare system, but they do like their own doctor, and most of the 84 percent of Americans who have health insurance believe they're going to get good care if they become ill. Therefore, despite the fact that they know what the problems are, they are reluctant to see significant changes in their personal situation—unless of course they become ill and find out they really don't have the health insurance they thought they did.

Therefore, health reformers must assure Americans who already have insurance that our prescription for change will secure their access to coverage. Reform isn't just about covering the uninsured or lowering costs over the long term. Reform will protect Americans and their families from a medical or financial catastrophe and preserve the care they already receive, provide them more coverage options, and strengthen the doctor–patient relationship.

The debate also needs to be framed around the economic impact that rising healthcare costs have on American jobs. As I write in chapter 2, health reform is business reform.

And the debate also needs to be framed in terms of the plight of the uninsured. As a nation, we are only as healthy as our sickest link. To lower our healthcare spending and really reorient the system away from just treating sickness and toward preventing illness, we have to insure every American.

The Debate Has Focused Erroneously on the British Model

The political fault lines in the development of a comprehensive healthcare program are the result of history. Every system devised by human beings has built on that which has come before it. In Europe, the massive destruction of infrastructure, including healthcare infrastructure, during World War II ushered in reform with a heavy government hand. As Atul Gawande described in *The New Yorker*, the war compelled the British government "to provide free hospital treatment for civilian casualties, as well as for combatants." Financial responsibility for all this healthcare fell largely on the government, a situation that only intensified after the Blitz of September 1940, which devastated medical infrastructure. Government programs were intended as temporary fixes, but, according to Gawande, "the war destroyed the status quo for patients, doctors, and hospitals alike. Moreover, the new system proved better than the old."

As a result, Gawande explains, the universal coverage that "emerged in Britain was not the product of socialist ideology or a deliberate policy process in which all the theoretical options were weighed. It was, instead, an almost conservative creation: a program that built on a tested, practical means of providing adequate health care for everyone, while protecting the existing services that people depended upon every day."

America and other industrialized nations haven't chosen to forgo the British system because it didn't work. Rather, other nations didn't adopt the British model because they constructed their universal healthcare under different circumstances. First of all, in this country, we did not see the destruction and depravation which was widespread in Europe during World War II.

It is no coincidence that Canada, Australia, and New Zealand developed their systems significantly later than the Europeans did, since they, like the United States, did not have massive homeland privation and destruction to cope with as a result of the war. Even in Europe, though, healthcare systems, while having in common a high degree of government involvement, have evolved very differently based on what happened before the war. The German and Dutch systems, for instance, feature significantly more decentralization and less government involvement than, say, their French and British counterparts.

In America, healthcare reformers will have to embrace reform that builds on the patchwork of private insurance networks and employer-based healthcare that developed in the wake of World

War II wage restraints. In other words, rather than completely dismantling the existing healthcare institutions and transferring all Americans into a new system, reformers must ensure care continuity—building on what works, while fixing what's broken.

Special-Interest Groups Defend the Status Quo

As you'll see in chapter 10, another major reason reform is so hard to pass is the lobbying done by powerful special interests, whose knee-jerk reaction is to defend the status quo. Until now these interest groups have included pharmaceutical companies; doctors, in the form of professional organizations such as the American Medical Association; health insurance companies; and employers, who, while suffering under the burden of rapidly increasing costs, have been innately suspicious of greater government involvement in regulation of the healthcare industry. Hospitals, which want as much autonomy as possible, fear payment reforms that could drive down their revenue, and ancillary medical supply groups and other providers want as much independence from government regulation as possible. During President Clinton's attempt to reform the healthcare system, this medical-industrial complex successfully convinced the American people that Clinton's reforms would jeopardize their existing coverage.

These groups have successfully defeated almost all past reform efforts. Their coalition has been remarkably effective. In the early 1990s, now Secretary of State Hillary Clinton, as first lady, led a task force to revamp the healthcare system. The group, through a somewhat opaque process, developed a very complicated proposal. The proposed new system itself made sense and offered the average American more choice of physicians and insurance plans than the existing system (the system we have today), but it suffered from two weaknesses. The first was that it was hard to understand. The second was that it was put together behind closed doors in a way that played into the hands of its opponents.

The attacks that followed became a political legend. Special-interest groups defined Clinton's plan before the administration could define it itself, despite the public's overwhelming support for greater government involvement in healthcare.

The insurance industry sponsored a series of "Harry and Louise" ads, falsely claiming that President Clinton's efforts to reform the healthcare system would undermine existing coverage and leave healthcare decisions in the hands of government bureaucrats. One ad was set "sometime in the future" and depicted actors Harry Johnson and Louise Claire Clark sitting at a kitchen table, shuffling through medical bills. "This was covered under our old plan," Louise reminds Harry. "Oh yeah, that was a good one, wasn't it," he recalls nostalgically. Then an ominous announcer's voice reminds viewers, "Things are changing, and not all for the better. The government may force us to pick from a few health-care plans designed by government bureaucrats." Louise: "Having choices we don't like is no choice at all." Harry: "They choose." Louise: "We lose."

The assumptions behind the ads—that people would no longer be able to choose their doctors, that there would be enormous amounts of paperwork, that the government would run every-thing—were disingenuous. But the campaign successfully played on the fears of the American people, who couldn't understand what the real plan said because it was so complicated. Harry and Louise, portrayed as quintessential Americans, pleasantly and plaintively threw out "facts" about the proposed plan that simply were not true. But they did help opponents of the Clinton plan sow doubts, many of them unfounded, about what might be in the plan.

In 1993, when the Clinton plan was under consideration, most Americans believed that the government must reform the health-care system. According to one poll, **83 percent of Americans** believed that it was very important that any healthcare reform plan made sure all Americans were covered. Sixty-one percent said they were willing to pay higher taxes to achieve this goal, and more than half said they were "willing to have the Government require employers to pay most of the health insurance premiums to cover their workers."

Americans Fear Change but Want Improvements

Americans remain concerned sixteen years later. Today 62 percent of voters say the economic crisis makes it more important than ever to take on healthcare reform, but many Americans are still nervous that healthcare overhaul may actually worsen their coverage. According to the pollsters, voters are as anxious about changing the healthcare system as they are hopeful that change would help them personally. As healthcare reform veteran Chris Jennings explains, "When it comes to health reform, fear beats hope. In the past, this has meant that nothing gets done."

Since 1948, reformers have failed to recognize that Americans like the kind of healthcare they get, *if* they have it available to them. The problem is not in convincing the American people that we need reform; they've heard that message before and they overwhelmingly agree with it.

The real goal, this time, is to do a better job in mobilizing that public support into action for change. It's about getting all the troops behind a proposal that lowers costs, expands coverage, and gives Americans the choice of keeping their current coverage or enrolling in a new public or private health insurance plan. And it's also about flipping anxiety about reform into anxiety about inaction. There is a famous saying in the Vermont legislature: "When in doubt, vote no." Fortunately, when it comes to healthcare, voting no is no longer an option. This time, the debate about health insurance will be different.

The Default Can No Longer Be "No"

Today, unlike the mid-1990s, most Americans recognize that the status quo is no longer the default option. The insured can now sympathize with their uninsured brethren. Anytime there is a major recession, millions of middle-class Americans lose their health insurance because they lose their jobs. As of this publication, employers have shed 5.7 million jobs since December 2007. Approximately 2.4 million workers have lost the health coverage their jobs provided, and more than 1 million workers lost health coverage in the first three months of 2009. In March 2009 alone, more than 320,000 Americans lost their employer-provided health insurance, which amounts to approximately 10,680 workers a day.

In an employer-based system, when you lose your job you lose your health insurance. So-called COBRA payments, which permit people who have lost jobs with larger employers to continue on their insurance plans for eighteen months, are unrealistically expensive. They range in price from $300 a month for those in their midtwenties who are single with no dependents to payments of $1,100 to $1,200 a month for middle-aged people with families. These expenses are prohibitive, since the people who have lost their jobs often have no resources.

Even more agonizing is the dilemma faced by families that have a small amount of resources. The usual scenario is to watch them slowly exhaust their savings and their home equity, if they can get a loan—unlikely under such circumstances— and then begin to make the devastating choices among paying the mortgage, paying for health insurance, adequately feeding their children, and perhaps giving up dreams of college for their children.

Of course, the number of people afraid of being laid off and losing their health insurance is greater than the number that actually loses coverage. But more and more Americans are vicariously experiencing the consequences of losing employer-based coverage or purchasing high-deductible plans through seeing the suffering of their friends and neighbors or through media accounts that detail the risks of inadequate insurance.

New Allies for the Next Congressional Debate on Healthcare Reform

Personally, I'm most proud of the growing support for reform from the provider community.

A majority of primary care physicians, and an increasing number of specialists, now believe that a single payer, like Medicare, will simplify their practices and improve quality of care. While the Medicare bureaucracy is no less complicated today than it was sixteen years ago, the proliferation of regulation and meddling by private insurance companies is leading some doctors to embrace reform. Today medical providers spend an inordinate amount of money responding to insurance company queries, settling billing disputes, and reacting to denied-treatment letters.

It would be far easier for physicians, particularly those in private practice, to have a single form to fill out, preferably on a universal electronic records system, created by people who actually listen to doctors before they design the system. This would change the equation dramatically in the practice of medicine. It is not uncommon in a hospital today to have billing offices that are nearly the size of the active medical staff. I have written previously about how much bureaucracy there is in insurance companies. The same is true of hospitals, whether for-profit or nonprofit. In order to maximize their revenue in an increasingly complicated and opaque, and in many cases frankly dishonest, profit-oriented atmosphere, hospitals must resort to clever coding that maximizes revenue and fill out multiple insurance forms. They must deal with frequent rejections by insurance companies based on technicalities. They must cope with oversights by third parties who have never seen the patient and often have no medical or nursing degrees. All of this takes money. A lot of money. This what American taxpayers and insurance rate payers are now handing over.

Similarly, hospitals, which opposed the Clinton plan, will be divided. The for-profit hospital system, which according to *The New England Journal of Medicine* does not provide care nearly as good as that found in nonprofit hospital systems, will likely oppose any attempt by government to increase oversight and payment. Institutions will be afraid that downward pressure exercised by a public health insurance option will cut into their profits and return on equity. A for-profit company has fiduciary responsibility to its shareholders, as conservative economist Milton Friedman often pointed out. They are in a business, however, that provides a public good—in fact, a public necessity. So they must provide the public necessity—but do so while minimizing the cost of care—in order to make ever-increasing quarterly returns and cause their stock to rise on Wall Street.

The nonprofit hospital system will likely be ambivalent about the plan. The nonprofit system, in particular, has been badly squeezed by the private insurance companies. In many cases, small, rural, and inner-city hospitals have either experienced bankruptcies or had to dramatically scale back. This is partly due to cutbacks on public reimbursements by governors and Congress trying to save money on healthcare costs. It is also due to increasing refusal by private health insurance companies to pay for adequate reimbursement for primary care providers—who are essential particularly for inner-city and rural delivery of care. The nonprofit hospital system will likely be grateful that many of their clients who now can pay nothing for health insurance will be able to pay for treatment when they join the ranks of insured Americans.

So in this new attempt at health reform, we see a different set of allies. The American Medical Association, in March 2009, put out a very equivocal and neutral statement after hearing from Henry Waxman, chairman of the committee in the House, which will oversee much of the House's effort to reform health-care. AMA president Nancy Nielsen said, "Health care reform should include a public and private mix of insurance. Let's give individuals choice so they can select appropriate coverage for themselves and their families." That statement is compatible with what President Obama's healthcare plan does. During the fight over the Clinton plan sixteen years ago, such a statement from the AMA would have been unthinkable. In fact, it looks like the only ally the health insurance industry will have in this fight is the right-wing ideological Republican Party. Many Republicans still oppose any kind of increasing public role for the same reasons they did in the mid-1990s. They just don't like government.

While the coffers and skills of the lobbyists for private health insurance companies should never be underestimated, they should not be allowed to overcome the needs of the medical profession, hospitals, and, most importantly, the American people as we design a healthcare plan that works for everyone.

chapter ten

The Black Hats: Special Interests and Other Opposition

In the aftermath of President Obama's election, the health insurance industry declared its support for reforming the health-care system. Rather than attack President Obama's principles for reform, the insurance industry and the medical-industrial complex publicly embraced the president and the notion of change. Everyone expressed the need for reform, and nobody considered the status quo a viable second option. Yet while these interests have successfully co-opted the language of health reform, they have not embraced the real goal of healthcare reform: providing everyone with a choice of coverage.

Private Insurers

America's Health Insurance Plans, the lobbying arm of the insurance industry, led this somewhat agreeable chorus of special interests that had so loudly protested President Clinton's health reform efforts just sixteen years earlier. Under the leadership of the very capable Karen Ignagni, AHIP embarked on a so-called listening tour around the country and released its own principles for reform in December 2008.

"We're hoping that by offering these proposals early we can contribute to the discussions. . . . [We] wanted to play a leadership role and not shrink from the challenges of here and now," Ignagni announced at the National Press Club unveiling of the industry's "uniquely American proposal." In some ways, the AHIP proposal closely tracks Obama's healthcare principles, but it also undermines the goal of real healthcare reform. That is, in order to fend off competition from a public healthcare option, the industry presented a set of minor policy changes wrapped in the flag of healthcare reform. While AHIP argues that it is ready to compromise on key issues, reading the fine print reveals otherwise.

The plan builds on the current employer-based system, expands Medicaid to establish a "clear, simple, transparent income test" in which everyone above 100 percent of the Federal Poverty Level (FPL) is eligible for coverage, requires the federal government to subsidize coverage on a sliding scale, guarantees coverage to everyone—so long as everyone is required to purchase health insurance coverage—and encourages Congress to set a target of a 30 percent reduction in future growth of healthcare expenditures. It also calls for an independent commission to look at variations in practice patterns, cost shifting, supply patterns, and cost consolidation, as well as laying out a road map to achieving the national target.

In March, AHIP and the Blue Cross Blue Shield Association formally announced that the insurance industry would be willing to charge every American the same price for health insurance coverage in the individual insurance market if the government protected its market monopoly, required all Americans to purchase their insurance product, and held off on the new public health option. "We believe that we could guarantee issue coverage with no pre-existing condition exclusions and phase out the practice of varying premiums based on health status in the individual market," the industry wrote in a letter to Congress. "While we support transitioning to a reformed system in which health-status-based rating is no longer used, rating flexibility based on age, geography, family size, and benefit design is needed to maintain affordability."

The media amplified their message. *The New York Times*, *USA Today*, and *The Washington Post* framed AHIP's announcement as an unprecedented concession—the industry coming to the table in good faith to reform the healthcare system and save the American worker from skyrocketing healthcare costs. "Tuesday's proposal marked one of the first concrete steps forward in the process," *USA Today* gushed. The letter "is the latest move by health insurers to position themselves as constructive participants, rather than obstacles, in the debate over how to overhaul the U.S. health-care system," *The Wall Street Journal* observed.

But it's unclear what exactly AHIP is conceding. For one, the industry made very similar "concessions" in December 1992, promising to "provide the standard package 'regardless of a person's medical history'" and to work with the government to "stabilize health-care prices" if everyone was required to purchase insurance. This latest proposal is, for the most part, just a regurgitation of past efforts—proposals the industry rejected once the administration proposed an actual plan. AHIP has embraced a modified form of community rating, but the industry did not rule out charging different rates "based on age, geography, family size, and benefit design." That means that a person in a wealthier area (who is generally healthier) could be charged a lower price than someone from the inner city (and in poorer health).

AHIP is all for "affordable" coverage on the government's dime. That is, it wants the government to issue tax credits and cap total health expenditures for lower-income individuals to protect Americans from bankruptcy. The plan calls on the government to ensure affordability while protecting industry profits. The health insurance industry also argues that we should set a target for reducing further growth. In fact, that target has been set for years with all sorts of ineffective government edicts, and still the costs of private health insurance continue to grow at two to three times the rate of inflation.

And this time, AHIP has nothing to lose. It's asking the

government to protect and even increase its monopoly on providing insurance to Americans under sixty-five and to strengthen safety-net programs that would siphon off the poorest (read: sickest) Americans. If the private insurance sector really wants to compete with the government, it should not need a subsidy to do so. Again, industries have no constitutional right to a subsidy or to maintain inefficiencies. There is, however, a fiduciary duty of Congress to provide the best services at the lowest price to the American taxpayers.

AHIP insists that private insurers would be unable to fairly compete with a Medicare-like public plan that did not have the capital reserves of private insurers or the ability to build networks of providers. The public plan would crowd out private insurers, underpay medical providers, and pass those costs to consumers in the form of higher premiums.

But why should we concern ourselves about the financial stability of private insurers? Health reform isn't about protecting private industry; it's about lowering healthcare costs and ensuring that every American has choice in affordable coverage. Moreover, the industry's sense of fair competition is itself unfair. The industry does not want a new public health insurance plan to have any inherent advantages, but it's insisting that private insurers preserve their advantage to create provider networks and enter or exit markets as they wish. As one Democratic senator pointed out during a recent Senate Finance Committee panel on healthcare coverage options, "It's sort of as if you're saying well, the public advantages we should get rid of, but the private advantages we should keep. Let them compete."

Indeed, while the industry is seeking to clone the public model into a private plan, most public plan advocates envision a system in which private and public plans complement each other and each plan uses its inherent advantages to offer Americans a real choice of coverage. So, while the public plan does not have explicit capital reserves like private plans, it will not be able to enter and exit different markets as most private plans could. The public plan may not have different networks of providers, but it could be a reliable source of coverage that contracts with any provider willing to accept its reimbursement rates (like Medicare). In other words, public and private plans are inherently different and will use those differences to compete and attract beneficiaries.

Moreover, the industry's argument that the public plan's lower rates of provider reimbursement to hospitals and doctors would shift the cost difference onto Americans with private insurance assumes that private plans are always right in setting reimbursement rates. As it turns out, however, "high payments from private insurers do not result from low payments for Medicare patients." As one recent Medicare Payment Advisory Commission (MedPAC) study found, "Claims of extensive cost shifting imply that hospital costs are largely fixed and that it is hospitals in the worst financial state that will have the greatest need and incentive to shift costs onto private payers due to low Medicare payment." But MedPAC concluded that "it is the most financially pressured hospitals that are most efficient and thus capable of earning money on Medicare patients." In other words, overpayments by private insurers to healthcare providers drives up healthcare costs.

I argue that choice is an endemic part of the American system. All the systems of healthcare in the industrialized world that are universal have some component of private insurance. That will continue under the system that President Obama suggested on the campaign trail. The American people have a right to an option should they be dissatisfied with the public plan. The Dutch people have such an option, as do the British, the Germans, and others. All have systems in which public insurance plays a significant role. There ought never be an exclusive right for private insurance companies to charge enormous prices, to operate inefficiently, and to exhibit the behavior they so frequently have in cutting healthcare to sick people, refusing to insure people who take certain medications or have certain diseases, and passing out contracts that are so difficult to read that people often think they have insurance for particular conditions when, in fact, they don't.

The opponents of healthcare reform specialize in self-serving suggestions. They believe the federal government should subsidize their product and require every American to purchase private coverage. While academics can argue about the necessity of mandating coverage, for-profit health insurance companies will benefit by having more people sign up for their expensive products.

Pharmaceutical Companies

Pharmaceutical companies will also oppose Americans' right to choose a public health insurance option. The major concern that drug companies have is whether or not the government will use their huge purchasing power to ratchet down prices. While we can debate whether this is a good idea or not, it's not the focus of the push toward real reform in healthcare.

Small Business

Another group that has opposed past healthcare reform efforts is the National Federation of Independent Business. Opposition by health insurance companies is understandable; they fear for their profits because of their inability to be as efficient as the public health insurance option will be. The opposition by NFIB, which has long been associated with right-wing causes, is far more perplexing. As I pointed out in chapter 2—with the story of my meeting with a trade association in Vermont—small business owners are reflexively conservative. But they will benefit more than any other segment of the business sector if the president's plan is adopted.

Both Democrats and Republicans pound their chests during every campaign season, proclaiming what they will do for small businesses. The truth is, over the last twenty years, neither party has done very much for small business at all. Small firms must shoulder more risk than any other sector of American entrepreneurship, but they also create 80 percent of all new jobs in our country. One of the biggest problems they face is difficulty retaining workers because it is so hard for them to bear the expense of healthcare plans that generally are much more expensive or have fewer benefits than plans offered by large, well-established competitors. The Obama healthcare proposal says to these businesses, *We will take over supporting your employees' health insurance. We will give you a refundable tax credit of up to 50 percent on premiums paid by you on behalf of your employees.* Small businesses would also have the option of enrolling their employees in the new public healthcare program or purchasing coverage from a private insurance company within the new insurance exchange. Very small businesses will be exempt from any responsibility for an employee's health insurance. That will be paid for solely by the employee and a government subsidy based on the employee's income.

The same conservatives who claim they want to help small business are opposed to the subsidy of small businesses through this plan. It is an extraordinary anomaly to see the National Federation of Independent Business, which claims to represent small business in Congress, fighting against a plan that could do so much for its own membership. There is no reason we shouldn't help our small businesses. Entrepreneurs create jobs in huge numbers relative to the rest of our economy. We have lost hundreds of thousands of jobs every month in the last year or so. We are in desperate need of more, and the quickest way to get them is to make it easier for small businesses to do business. There is no greater help the federal government could implement directly and in a short period of time than to enact the president's plan, which offers small businesses the option of enrolling their workers in an efficient public health insurance option. This is the best way to restore our economic prosperity and allow more Americans the opportunity to live out the American dream.

Big Business

These lobbying groups, the for-profit health insurance industry and the National Federation of Independent Business, are, along with the U.S. Chamber of Commerce, among the most ruthless in Washington. They have vast amounts of money, which they deploy in ads that are far from truthful. They use unconscionable scare tactics to influence American voters.

This time their task will be more difficult because the truth is very simple: You can keep what you have if you like it, or you can choose a government plan that may be more helpful.

During President Clinton's healthcare reform fight, the Business Roundtable—the lobbying arm of America's largest businesses—endorsed a rival plan that promised only access, not coverage. The rival proposal, sponsored by Representative Jim Cooper (D-TN), would have created insurance cooperatives for small businesses only, and it did not require businesses to pay 80 percent of employee insurance costs as the Clinton plan did. John Ong, chairman of the Roundtable, criticized the Clinton plan for creating "unfunded off-budget entitlement programs" and "price controls." Similarly, the Chamber of Commerce, after initially using the rhetoric of reform and supporting an employer mandate, reneged and decided that "our membership is not in support of the employer mandate approach." "The board is rejecting any form of employer mandate," chamber president Richard Lesher said.

Today most large companies have generally embraced the president's health principles, and I suspect that the chairmen of many corporate boards are currently debating the merits of Obama's approach. The truth is, most big businesses want to continue providing affordable coverage to their workers. They are a key stakeholder in the healthcare debate and, given the realities of our employer-based healthcare system, often use health benefits to attract and retain highly qualified employees. I believe that while most big businesses are wary of greater government involvement, lowering healthcare prices is the best way to help American businesses compete in the increasingly difficult international market.

I was in a recent discussion about the automobile industry with a group of economists, one of whom said, "Well, of course you know that General Motors is one of the largest health insurance companies in the world." That probably says more about the state of the automobile industry than anything else. Generally speaking, management doesn't do well managing industries in which it does not specialize. For General Motors, Ford, and Chrysler to do well, they need to make automobiles that Americans want to buy, not worry about keeping up with the ever-increasing costs of providing health insurance coverage.

Conservatives

During the early 1990s, under the leadership of Representative Newt Gingrich (R-GA) and Senator Bob Dole (R-KS) and bolstered by the ideological support of the Heritage Foundation, Cato Institute, and Manhattan Institute, Republicans successfully defeated President Clinton's health reform effort. Conservatives of all stripes argued that healthcare reform was "creeping socialism" or "big government," denied the existence of a healthcare crisis, or co-opted the term *reform* to push their own agendas and dilute support for a comprehensive solution to the nation's healthcare crisis.

Unfortunately, today's Republicans are no less inflammatory. Relying on a very similar playbook, conservatives are distorting progressive proposals in an effort to obstruct reform. In May 2009, GOP wordsmith Frank Luntz authored a new messaging memo defining the Republican rhetoric on healthcare reform. The memo, titled "The Language of Healthcare 2009," "is based on polling results and . . . captures not just what Americans want to see but exactly what they want to hear." The memo suggests "The Words That Work" and instructs that "from today forward, they should be used by everyone."

Luntz warns that "if the dynamic becomes 'President Obama is on the side of reform and Republicans are against it,' then the battle is lost and every word in this document is useless." The trouble is, the document is already useless. Because rather than challenging the tenets of American reform proposals, Luntz establishes a straw man argument against a nonexistent health plan. Buried amid the usual rhetoric about government-run healthcare is Luntz's predictable contradiction: He instructs Republicans to "be vocally and passionately on the side of REFORM" but then urges GOP lawmakers to misrepresent and obstruct any real chance of passing comprehensive legislation.

"Humanize your approach," but argue that healthcare reform "will result in delayed and potentially even denied treatment, procedures and/or medications." "Acknowledge the crisis" but ask your constituents "would you rather . . . 'pay the costs you pay today for the quality of care you currently receive,' OR 'Pay less for your care, but potentially have to wait weeks for tests and months for treatments you need.'"

In other words, say there is a crisis but then argue that healthcare reform would lead to "the government setting standards of care" and government "rationing care" and would "put the Washington bureaucrats in charge of health care." "This plays into more favorable Republican territory by protecting individual care while downplays the need for a comprehensive national plan," the memo states.

Readers are also instructed to conflate Obama's fairly moderate hybrid approach to reform (building on the current private-public system of delivering healthcare) with "denial horror stories from Canada & Co."

Focus on timeliness—"the plan put forward by the Democrats will deny people treatments they need and make them wait to get the treatments they are allowed to receive"—and argue that Republicans will provide "in a word, more: 'more access to more treatments and more doctors . . . with less interference from insurance companies and Washington politicians and special interests.'"

But that's the major problem with Luntz's memo: It tries to obstruct health reform by ignoring what Obama is actually offering. Instead, Luntz is attacking an easy extreme—what he wishes the Democrats were proposing—and pretending that the Republicans actually have some kind of healthcare solution (the memo instructs Republicans to focus on targeting waste, fraud, and abuse).

For their part, Republicans have no solution to the healthcare crisis. In fact, a recent article in Politico.com noted that the GOP is "stumbling" to find new ideas for reforming the healthcare system. "No Republicans leading the charge . . . have coalesced the party behind them," the article notes. "**Their message is still vague and unformed. Their natural allies among insurers, drug makers and doctors remain at the negotiating table with the Democrats.** So Republicans now worry the party has waited so long to figure out where it stands that it will make it harder to block what President Barack Obama is trying to do."

To the extent that Republicans are discussing healthcare, they're relying on trite McCain-campaign talking points and old hands from the 1990s. In other words, they've outsourced the conversation to attack dogs and relinquished the serious debate about how to lower costs, increase access, and improve quality.

The truth, and what the Politico.com article hints at, is that the GOP leadership has little understanding of health-care issues. In February 2009, House Republicans formed a study group to devise so-called free-market alternatives to President Obama's healthcare proposal. Minority Leader John Boehner (R-OH) tapped former GOP whip Representative Roy Blunt (R-MO) to lead the group of sixteen Republicans, including Representatives Michael Burgess (R-TX) and John Shadegg (R-AZ). "Through this working group, Republicans will develop real solutions to improve our health care system by putting patients before paperwork and frivolous lawsuits," Blunt promised. But at the group's first meeting, "members reviewed polling data and agreed to bring in a series of experts to discuss problems with the health care system and potential solutions." As of this writing, the Republicans have yet to embrace a healthcare solution or properly diagnose the cause of the healthcare crisis.

In April, the Health Policy Consensus Group, headed by the conservative Galen Institute, published "a vision for consumer-driven health care reform" that focuses on tax breaks for health-care and giving Americans "control" over their healthcare dollars. Senator John McCain (R-AZ) had proposed a similar plan during the presidential campaign, but he never convinced Americans to abandon their employer-provided insurance for the promise of cheaper coverage in the individual market. Part of the problem rests in the fallacy of the theory; the rest, in the burden of experience. After all, Americans are routinely denied coverage in the unregulated individual health insurance market, and small businesses are "frequently finding health policies too expensive and are dropping coverage, sending even more people shopping for insurance." Healthy Americans who do find coverage enroll in bare-bones plans that offer little substantive protection.

As *The Miami Herald* recently reported, insurers deny coverage for patients with "diabetes, hepatitis C, multiple sclerosis, schizophrenia, quadriplegia, Parkinson's disease and AIDS/HIV." Moreover, "some insurers will automatically reject applicants who are using certain prescription drugs. Wellpoint denies anyone who within the past year has taken Abilify and Zyprexa for mental disorders as well as Neupogen, which is used to treat the side effects of chemotherapy. Vista lists the anticoagulant warfarin and the pain medication OxyContin. Both companies list insulin."

And why not? Competition without meaningful regulations incentivizes companies to offer insurance to only the healthiest Americans. How else could they beat the insurer across the street? Offering coverage to sicker Americans would attract a sicker pool of enrollees and serve as a competitive disadvantage. In fact, free-market healthcare fits the definition of a failed market. A market fails when these conditions exist:

- *A monopoly, which occurs if a single buyer or seller can exert significant influence over prices or output.* In healthcare, "insurer and hospital markets are increasingly dominated by large insurers and provider systems," an Urban Institute report points out. "The increased concentration has made it difficult for the nation to reap the benefits usually associated with competitive markets."
- *Negative externalities, which occur if the market does not take into account the impact of an economic activity on outsiders.* In the Wild West environment of the individual health marketplace, companies leave the sickest patients without coverage. Healthcare costs

increase for everyone when patients are forced to forgo
early and appropriate care or to visit the emergency
room once a condition becomes unbearable.

- *Asymmetric information, which occurs when one party
  has more or better information than the other party.*
  Americans looking for coverage in the individual
  market have no way of comparing different policies
  and rarely know what the plans actually cover.

Conservative health proposals double down on this broken
marketplace. They: (1) eliminate the employer tax exemption for health benefits, (2) provide everyone with a refundable tax credit to go out and purchase individual coverage, and
(3) loosen the already lax insurer regulations. The results are
predictable. Not only will Americans with preexisting conditions go without coverage—or, at best, be offered very expensive
plans—but as healthy Americans with bare-bones policies fall
ill, they'll discover that their insurer has little enthusiasm for
paying claims.

Conservatives may no longer deny the existence of a healthcare
crisis, but they sure do misdiagnose the causes of rising healthcare costs. Blunt, for instance, promised that "Republicans will
develop real solutions to improve our health care system by
putting patients before paperwork and frivolous lawsuits." But to
identify "real solutions," we must first properly diagnose the problem. Blunt's argument that "frivolous lawsuits" are significantly
driving up healthcare costs misses the point entirely.

The total cost of malpractice constitutes just 0.46 percent
of total healthcare expenditures, and settlements have grown
modestly with inflation. While approximately 98,000 people die
each year from negligent treatment, a mere 2 percent sue their
physicians. As health policy analyst Maggie Mahar observed,
"A very small group of doctors are losing or settling malprac-

tice lawsuits, but they are losing big." Between 1990 and 2002, "5.2 percent of doctors were responsible for 55 percent" of all malpractice payouts. The increasing costs of malpractice insurance premiums are hurting doctors, but they're not the real causes of our growing healthcare bill. In reality, the longer Republicans obscure the real issues and obstruct reform efforts, the higher the costs will rise.

— part four —

SHATTERING HEALTHCARE MYTHS

chapter eleven

Healthcare Reform Is Not a New Idea

America's employer-based healthcare system formed in response to the anti-inflationary atmosphere during and shortly after World War II. Employers, in many cases, were discouraged or forbidden to give raises to their employees during those years. So, to sweeten the pot for the employees they wanted to retain, they seized upon the idea of giving healthcare benefits, which did not count as wages. The federal government encouraged this and, to make it more attractive, eventually exempted health insurance from taxation. This is why, over the years, healthcare became a fringe benefit paid for by the business sector.

Efforts to reform this system began sixty years ago when President Harry Truman, seeing the direction every other industrialized democracy in the world was going, and following the example of postwar Europe, announced that we, too, should embark on a system of universal healthcare coverage, in which the government could be the principal coordinator, if not payer, of healthcare coverage.

Since that time, there have been multiple attempts to change our system. Most efforts have built on our public-private hybrid model of delivering care. Presidents Carter and Clinton, for instance, both tried, without effect, to make changes in our system so that every American would have what every European has—universal access to healthcare.

Public Healthcare Really Began in the 1960s

The only successful attempt at major reform occurred in 1965, when President Lyndon Johnson signed legislation establishing Medicare and Medicaid. Medicare, which now covers every American over sixty-five, and Medicaid, which insures tens of millions of low-income Americans, particularly children, are examples of "government-run single payers."

Yet in the post-Goldwater era, the Republican Party strongly denounced Medicaid and Medicare as "socialized medicine." In one well-known 1961 advertisement, Ronald Reagan—then a Republican pitchman—urged his listeners to oppose the growing menace of socialized medicine, arguing that Medicare legislation would lead to national socialism. If Medicare was passed, he warned, "one of these days, you and I are going to spend our sunset years telling our children and our children's children what it once was like in America, when men were free."

Today, Medicare is one of the most extraordinary programs ever devised in America. Together with Social Security, it changed the lives of people over sixty-five in America. In the 1930s, to be an American over the age of sixty-five was to be a member of the poorest age group in the country. Now most seniors find themselves in the middle class of America, and senior poverty, while it exists, is a tiny fraction of what it once was. Social Security and Medicare are the two reasons that this is possible.

In that light, it is ironic that today—deep in the debate over health insurance—the words *socialized medicine* are still on the lips of many Republican senators and House members. They are still complaining, despite the success of our "socialized" programs. But the opportunity for real reform is back. Once again, as in 1965, Democrats have a large majority in the House and the Senate and control the White House. Once again, exactly as happened forty-five years ago, the Republicans have signaled that they have no intention of having the government involved in healthcare any more than it already is. And once again it seems likely that the Democrats will have to take both the leadership and complete responsibility for making this change in response to a resounding *no* from virtually every Republican in Congress.

The Changing Debate: From Covering the Uninsured to Controlling Costs

By the 1970s, the healthcare system was inflicting enormous costs on the American economy. Medical inflation and medical costs began to take center stage in the debate over healthcare reform, despite the drumbeat from the center left, which still advocated for expanding access to care for the uninsured.

By the end of that decade, hospitals were pushing to keep pace with ever-more-advanced care options, purchasing costly equipment and undertaking costly expansions. A wide variety of reform efforts had begun, in both the private and public sectors. Review programs were launched for proposed new hospitals and equipment, to make sure the need was justified before the expense was incurred. But even so, hospitals were unable to bend the upward curve of growing costs.

Eventually, insurance companies began to change the fine print in their plans, dropping coverage for preexisting conditions or refusing to pay for costly new illnesses. Their goal was to limit their risk and their outlay, and to intimidate physicians. Bureaucratic second-guessing became the norm within both private insurance companies and public healthcare. Both arenas hired people—many of whom had no medical background or had rarely seen patients—to review the procedures and medications prescribed by a patient's physician. Even though they had no expertise to make judgment calls on patients' needs, these case reviewers were essentially rationing care.

As the 1980s gave way to the 1990s, the imperative of covering all Americans and the desire to begin to restrain the extraordinary and prolonged inflationary costs of medical care received equal billing.

Despite all these efforts, healthcare costs have continued to rise for roughly thirty years at a rate between 200 and 300 percent of inflation. Today the percentage of our gross domestic product spent on healthcare is 17 percent. Most European nations with comprehensive universal healthcare programs spend between 6 and 10 percent of their gross domestic product on healthcare.

New Incentive for Reform

Now there is a new impetus to reform healthcare. The extraordinarily inflationary growth of healthcare over the past forty years has finally awakened the business community. So this round of healthcare reform will focus on three things:

- The corrosive effect of increasing healthcare costs on our ability to compete nationally to create and retain American jobs.
- The fact that many Americans with health insurance are essentially uninsured.
- The fact that, to our national disgrace, on average 16 percent of Americans have no health insurance—a figure that rises to 25 percent in states like Texas.

Reform of our healthcare system will be a tall order, and each of these problems needs to be addressed.

— chapter twelve —

How Do Other Countries Do It?

All other industrialized European and North American nations already provide health coverage to all their citizens. Since we spend about 6.1 percent more than the average of other industrialized countries on healthcare costs while leaving approximately 16 percent of our population without any form of health insurance, our global neighbors can offer valuable lessons for how to cover everyone and pay less for coverage.

This chapter asks: What can we learn from the experiences of different countries, and how can we apply their best practices to our healthcare reforms?

France

Most progressive healthcare advocates view France as the best hope for reform. The World Health Organization ranks the French healthcare system as the best in the world. In 1945, President Charles de Gaulle revamped a healthcare system that had been devastated by the war, building on the existing employer-based system. Today the French provide all of their citizens with standard health insurance benefits and few waiting lists. As a result, France has the highest level of satisfaction with healthcare among all European countries.

So what's their secret? Well, it's simple enough. Care is distributed through large occupation-based funds—alliances of professional groups—that are overseen by the government (it sets reimbursement fees with physicians and establishes premiums) and financed through taxes and general government revenues.

French citizens pay a substantial amount in cost sharing, but the government limits every individual's out-of-pocket expenses and keeps a list of approximately thirty chronic conditions that are exempt from any additional payments. This way, patients with hard-to-manage chronic conditions aren't penalized and don't avoid preventive care that could head off future medical complications (and increased costs).

Anyone can see any doctor at any time, without a referral or gatekeeper, and some 92 percent of French residents purchase complementary private insurance to pay for additional fees to access providers that may not accept the government-established fee schedules.

The French do have less access to some medical technologies, but that doesn't mean that they experience worse health outcomes. In fact, one recent study "comparing care in Manhattan and Paris found the care in Paris to be better largely because the Parisians have better access to routine and effective primary care—which is typical in universal health insurance systems."

The French rely on both private and public systems to provide all of their citizens with healthcare services. Open access to primary care and an emphasis on chronic care management keeps costs down (the French spend only 11 percent of their GDP on healthcare) and generates better health outcomes. The system preserves patient choice and allows private industry to fill an important niche, but government-established reimbursement rates and cost sharing may be more government control than we're used to.

Switzerland

This isn't the case in Switzerland. Before 1994, Switzerland had a healthcare system a lot like ours. The Swiss bought health insurance through their employer, insurance was voluntary, and many people found themselves excluded from coverage for all kinds of preexisting conditions, like asthma or cancer. Insurers would cherry-pick the healthiest individuals and leave the rest without health coverage.

As in America, Switzerland had its own share of special interests. Big insurance companies and drug companies dominated the political landscape, and when reformers like Ruth Dreifuss— health minister of the left-leaning Social Democratic Party— started talking about enacting reforms that would guarantee everyone access to health insurance, private industry complained that they would be forced out of business.

But in 1995, Dreifuss successfully spearheaded a referendum to reform the healthcare system. Everyone had to purchase healthcare coverage; insurers could no longer enroll only the healthiest individuals or make a profit on basic care. The government provided subsides to the poor and restructured the insurance industry in the same way that President Clinton had proposed in 1993.

Insurers compete for enrollees within a regulated exchange and offer everyone who applies the same standard benefits package. The policies are community rated, meaning the premiums of healthy people subsidize the care of unhealthy people.

Greater regulation of insurers has not run the industry out of business. To the contrary. Since they can no longer charge sicker people higher premiums or offer porous policies that exclude coverage for certain critical conditions, insurers try to attract enrollees by competing on price—varying the level of deductibles and co-payments. Insurers negotiate directly with providers and try to obtain the best possible price.

Still, the system is far from perfect. Since citizens are exposed to the full cost of health insurance—an employer does not help subsidize coverage, for instance—they have much higher out-of-pocket costs than we currently do and nationally spend 11.5 percent of the GDP on healthcare, the second highest in the world. The Swiss do demonstrate that managed competition among insurers can lower prices while preserving the role of private industry.

Netherlands

The Dutch, who recently reformed their healthcare system, adopted a similar scheme. All Dutch citizens are required to purchase health insurance from a menu of forty-two private insurance companies. The Health Ministry sets premiums, but insurance companies can compete by offering different deductibles, and some even offer rebates to policyholders who use only primary care services during the year. The Dutch are required to purchase only standard benefits, so more than 90 percent of the population also buys supplemental insurance. Insurers negotiate quality, quantity, and price of services with medical providers and require them to adhere to evidence-based guidelines of practice.

As in Switzerland, competition has lowered prices. According to one study, more competition among insurers has increased the purchasing power of Dutch households by 1.5 percent, and healthcare costs "have been growing at an annual rate of just 3 percent compared to more than 4.5 percent in the year before reforms."

It's important to note that there is no single model for universal healthcare and that every system developed through a series of historical accidents; every country has adopted a model that fits its own unique set of traditions and events.

Switzerland and the Netherlands provide all of their citizens with access to health insurance through a process of managed competition. Rather than directly paying for coverage—as in Canada and Britain—the government creates a framework within which insurers freely compete for enrollees. France, Germany, and Japan all operate under a managed competition arrangement but impose different cost-sharing rules and different subsidies for coverage and reimburse differently for medical services. Still, they all force insurers to play by a certain set of rules under which nobody slips through the cracks. Nobody is denied coverage. Nobody is swimming in medical debt. Everyone is covered and everyone pays less.

Germany

It is widely acknowledged that the first national healthcare system was enacted in Germany, in 1883, under Chancellor Otto von Bismarck. The German system has evolved over the years to cover 90 percent of all Germans with public money, and only some are required to purchase insurance. Citizens with incomes under $60,000 have to enroll in one of 240 different sickness funds; richer citizens can opt out and purchase private insurance.

Still, approximately 75 percent remain in the sickness funds. And why shouldn't they? The standard benefits package is fairly comprehensive and includes "physicians, hospital and chronic care, diagnostic tests, preventive care, prescription drugs, and parts of dental care." Sickness funds even pay "to those who cannot work due to illness, ranging from 70 to 90 percent of the patient's last gross salary for up to 78 weeks."

The government seeds the funds through a payroll tax split between the employer and the employee, but the lowest-wage workers are entirely funded by the government and essentially receive free care, with some co-payments. As workers rise on the wage scale, the tax burden increases, so the more prosperous contribute more through taxes.

As in Switzerland and the Netherlands, sickness funds are not allowed to make a profit on standard care. Instead, they compete to keep old customers and attract new ones, actively negotiate drug prices as well as standard prices with medical providers, and try to reduce administrative spending.

Despite the many successful foreign models for achieving universal health coverage through managed competition, Republicans are intent on portraying progressive healthcare proposals as imports from Britain or Canada, two systems that have little similarity to reforms now under consideration. Unlike France, Switzerland, or the Netherlands, Britain and Canada have single-payer systems in which a government body pays for the healthcare of all of its citizens through a global budget that allocates a certain portion of the nation's resources to healthcare and sets prices and reimbursement rates with providers.

Republicans are using this kind of system as a straw man to scare Americans into accepting the status quo. Reform the healthcare system and you will lose access to the coverage you already have, they argue. By amplifying the deficiencies of these two single-payer models and exaggerating their problems, Republicans are hoping to conflate President Obama's proposal with the long waiting lines and healthcare rationing.

In reality, President Obama has rejected a British/Canadian-like single-payer reform, and most policy makers are looking for a "uniquely American solution" that preserves the employer-sponsored system and creates a hybrid public-private partnership. In other words, American reforms would look a bit like the Swiss health system in which the government "leaves the provision of health care and health insurance in private hands" but creates a marketplace within which insurers can compete on price but can't avoid insuring the sickest patients.

Great Britain

The British system also evolved because of the privations of World War II and was established by conservative icon Winston Churchill. The expansion of the government's role was a necessity during the war, as large parts of the healthcare infrastructure were destroyed while healthcare needs increased significantly, often due to war-related injuries.

After the war, the ensuing labor government, capitalizing on the enormous popularity of the system that Churchill had brought in during the war, formalized universal healthcare. It was proposed in 1945 and enacted in 1948. I still remember living in England thirty-five years ago on an exchange scholarship and, as a student and a foreigner, getting new glasses for the equivalent of $5.

If you fall ill, you go to see your general practitioner, who acts as a gatekeeper to specialists. The National Health Service owns the vast majority of the country's hospitals and employs most doctors as salaried government workers. The average British primary care physician makes $220,000 per year. There is no malpractice problem. There are no insurance companies with hundreds of different forms. Everything is covered, from basic dental care to pharmaceutical needs. Eighty-seven percent of the expenditures are paid for by the government, 13 percent by the private sector.

The existence of waiting lists for nonessential care is a significant problem, and patients do experience delays in receiving treatment. But are British patients worse off than Americans, and do they have a healthcare system that delivers worse outcomes? The answer to both is no. As health blogger Ezra Klein explains, "In the case of ill health, they're actually in much better health than their American counterparts, though that's a function of lifestyle more than hospital choice. And in the case of health outcomes, it sort of depends. **You're probably better off getting**

your breast cancer treated in America and getting your diabetes treated in Britain. In the aggregate, however, the evidence
is fairly clear that the British are better off."

Canada

In Canada, the first healthcare system was developed in 1946
in the province of Saskatchewan. Unlike the German system,
in which some Germans get healthcare through their unions,
or so-called guilds, which are employer-related, there is no
relationship between employment and healthcare in Canada.
The government finances the system through a Medicaid-like
arrangement in which Canada's ten provinces and two territories jointly fund healthcare. Each province establishes provider
reimbursement rates; physicians work in private practice and are
paid on a fee-for-service basis. Everyone has access to care, but
Canadians do wait longer for services than most Americans. As
one study of waiting times for knee-replacement surgery in the
United States and Ontario found, the median waiting time for
an initial orthopedic consultation was two weeks in the United
States and four weeks in Ontario. Still, "overall satisfaction with
surgery was similar," the study concluded. Canadians also have
longer life expectancy, lower infant mortality rates, and lower
rates of obesity.

Waiting times are not ideal and even repugnant to most
Americans. We're used to getting the treatments we need when
we need them. No waiting, no lines, no lists. But our current
healthcare system has many of the same problems that British
and Canadian citizens experience. Those of us who can afford
good health insurance are not waiting for surgery, but for the 16
percent of the population that is uninsured and for the 25 million
Americans who don't have enough insurance, our healthcare
system denies, restricts, and rations care.

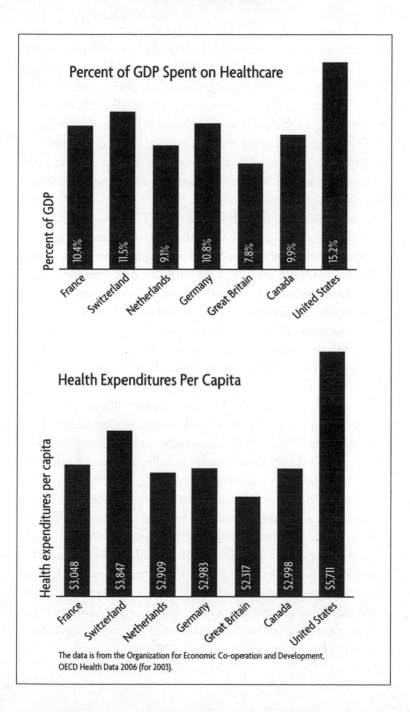

The data is from the Organization for Economic Co-operation and Development, OECD Health Data 2006 (for 2003).

Compared with other nations, the U.S healthcare system currently ranks last in all dimensions of a high-performance health system: quality, access, efficiency, equity, and healthy lives. Of course, if other countries can cover all of their citizens at a fraction of the cost that we spend denying care to millions, then studying the systems of other nations may offer a clue as to how to fix our own. One clue stands above the rest: Most capitalist countries don't leave healthcare to the open market or treat it like it's just another commodity.

As journalist T. R. Reid observed in his PBS documentary *Sick Around the World*, capitalist countries impose three basic limits on the free market: "First, insurance companies must accept everyone and can't make a profit on basic care. Second, everybody's mandated to buy insurance, and the government pays the premium for the poor. Third, doctors and hospitals have to accept one standard set of fixed prices."

But this isn't very foreign to American veterans who receive British-style healthcare from the VA, or for working Americans with insurance who have a German-like healthcare structure, or for Medicare recipients who have a Canadian-like system.

The truth is, so-called socialized medicine does exist in the United States. It has a very high satisfaction rate among its users and does a good job of keeping its enrollees in good health and maintaining low administrative costs.

The opposition to healthcare reform from Republicans, particularly the ideological right wing, is based on beliefs and ideology that are completely unsubstantiated by experiences in the rest of the world, or even here at home. The global systems discussed in this chapter may not be perfect, but they're a world away from our broken patchwork of healthcare insurers and providers. Our world neighbors are not advocating for adopting America's free-market approach. As we look to them for a better healthcare model, they look away from us.

— chapter thirteen —

Eleven Myths

As Congress considers healthcare reform, conservatives and their industry allies—so-called opponents of healthcare reform—will likely embark on a misinformation campaign about the consequences and implications of expanding access to affordable coverage. Here, debunked, are the right wing's most widely circulated myths about reform.

Myth 1: Healthcare reform will limit patient choice and lead to socialized medicine. The Republican alternative to President Obama's health reform efforts—the Patients' Choice Act—states, "The Federal government would run a health care system—or a public plan option—with the compassion of the IRS, the efficiency of the post office, and the incompetence of Katrina." The Cato Institute has published a brief asking "Does Barack Obama Support Socialized Medicine" before suggesting that "reasonable people can disagree over whether Obama's health plan would be good or bad. But to suggest that it is not a step toward socialized medicine is absurd." (Patients' Choice Act Summary, May 20, 2009; Cato Institute, October 7, 2008)

Reality: **Progressive reforms will provide more choice, not less.** Under progressive proposals, Americans will have the choice to keep the employer plan they currently have or buy an affordable plan from the national insurance exchange. Individuals and small businesses will be able to "compare private coverage options and a public plan and to purchase the policy that would work best for them." Moreover, to characterize Obama's healthcare as "socialized medicine" is itself "absurd." In contrast to Cato's rhetoric, socialized healthcare is "a system of health care delivery in which care is provided as a state-supported service." As Jeanne Lambrew, director of the Health and Human Services Office of Health Reform, points out, given Obama's reliance on private insurers and providers, accusations of socialism are "far from the truth." "Nonetheless, accusations of socialized medicine will likely continue to be raised about any reform proposal that is not based entirely on letting private insurance companies rule our health care system," she argues. (Baucus Health Plan, November 12, 2008; Center for American Progress, May 14, 2008)

Myth 2: Americans will lose their existing coverage. In a recent issue health brief, the Heritage Foundation charged that "the creation of a new public plan would result in millions of Americans losing their employment-based coverage." (Heritage Foundation, December 4, 2008)

Reality: **Progressive proposals strengthen the employer-based system by spreading the risk and cost of insurance.** A mandate for larger employers will encourage companies to continue providing coverage and will make healthcare more affordable by spreading the costs. A majority of large American employers would continue to provide coverage as a competitive benefit, while businesses with the fewest workers and the lowest wages would be exempt from the mandate and offered a new tax credit to purchase health insurance for their employees. (Baucus Health Plan, November 12, 2008)

Myth 3: The government will ration care. In his memo on healthcare, GOP wordsmith Frank Luntz says, "Nothing else turns people against the government takeover of healthcare [more] than the . . . expectation that it will result in delayed and potentially even denied treatment, procedures and/or medications." (The Language of Healthcare 2009, May 6, 2009)

Reality: **Government research that compares the clinical outcomes of alternative therapies will not ration care. They will inform doctors and patients on the most effective medical treatments and procedures.** Research into the comparative effectiveness of treatments can identify the procedures that provide the best results at the lowest cost. Currently, at least one-third of medical procedures have questionable benefits, according to the Rand Corporation. (Rand Corporation, 1998)

Myth 4: Affordable healthcare reform will create a government monopoly over healthcare. In her testimony to Congress, healthcare crisis denier Sally Pipes said, "My view is that the government plan will be priced lower than the private plans. The result will be 'crowding out' of the private plans and a fateful turn down the road to a Canadian style 'Medicaid for All' program." (Wonk Room, March 17, 2009)

Reality: **Progressive proposals for a public plan would create real choice and real competition, with all health plans focused on delivering better care at lower costs.** According to the Urban Institute, "The presence of a well-run public plan would constrain private spending, as the plans would have to compete on price." In fact, private insurers who "offer a superior product through high levels of efficiency, satisfaction in consumer preferences and ease of access to quality medical services" will thrive in a reformed market. The presence of a well-run and effective public plan will incentivize innovation in cost containment and service delivery. (Urban Institute, October 3, 2008)

Myth 5: A new public health plan will only drive up healthcare costs and increase premiums for Americans with private insurance. Karen Ignagni, the CEO of America's Health Insurance Plans, recently argued that "a new public program similar to

Medicare would exacerbate cost-shifting, which already adds $1,500, or 10 percent, to the average premium for a family of four." (*New York Times*, December 17, 2008)

Reality: **A public plan will contain costs, lower premiums, and give Americans a choice of health plans—public and private.** A recent analysis of the public option by the Institute for America's Future concluded that offering a new public insurance option to Americans who lack coverage would control healthcare costs and improve quality by providing an important benchmark for private insurance within a reformed healthcare framework. Universal coverage will reduce cost shifting by getting everybody covered and contain costs through investment in prevention, management of chronic care, twenty-first-century information technology, and research on and adoption of effective treatments. (Institute for America's Future, December 17, 2008)

Myth 6: Being uninsured is not a problem; it's people's own fault. During an interview with the independent student newspaper of Tufts University, former senator Bob Dole (R-KS) downplayed the number of Americans without health insurance. "However, 11 million of that total are illegal immigrants. Ten million more are people who can buy their own insurance. Finally, another 10 million are people your own age who think they are never going to get sick or hurt and are not vulnerable," Dole argued. (*Tufts Daily*, December 4, 2008)

Reality: **Americans are uninsured because they can't afford the high costs of insurance.** According to the Kaiser Family Foundation (KFF), most Americans who lack health insurance "come from working families and have low incomes." About two-thirds of the uninsured "are poor or near poor" and are "less likely to be offered employer-sponsored coverage or to be able to afford to purchase their own coverage." (Kaiser Family Foundation, October 15, 2008)

Myth 7: Illegal immigrants are driving the nation's uninsured problem. During the election, political strategist Dick Morris argued that "covering illegals adds dramatically to the cost of any program—and would encourage more folks to enter America illicitly." (Newsmax, July 21, 2008)

Reality: **Immigrants are not the primary factor driving the uninsured problem or rising healthcare costs.** As the Kaiser Family Foundation points out, while "non-citizens are much more likely to be uninsured than citizens" because of limited access to employer-based healthcare coverage and restrictions for public coverage, citizens still make up "the bulk of the uninsured." The majority (76 to 80 percent) of the growth in the number of uninsured from 2000 to 2006 occurred among citizens, not legal and undocumented noncitizens. Moreover, because noncitizens are much less likely than citizens to have a usual source of care, they have significantly lower per-capita healthcare expenditures than citizens and also are "generally restricted from enrolling in Medicaid and SCHIP." (Kaiser Family Foundation, March 11, 2008)

Myth 8: Healthcare reform won't save money. In a recent appearance on Fox News Channel, Fred Barnes of *The Weekly Standard* argued that affordable healthcare reform wouldn't save money or improve the quality of care. "In other words, we're going to insure all the uninsured, and they're going to have better healthcare. In other words, you're going to get a lot more for less. Now, does anybody who can tie his shoes believe that? I don't think so! Come on! That's ridiculous. We're going to save money. There's going to be a lot more for you, but it will cost a lot less," Barnes opined. (Wonk Room, December 12, 2008)

Reality: **If everyone had access to affordable healthcare and lifesaving preventive services, the system could better manage chronic diseases, end the cost shift from the uninsured to the insured, and improve efficiency.** A Families USA study found that uncompensated care for the uninsured contributes an average of $922 to family health insurance premiums. As Chris Jennings has pointed out, "If people go in and out of the system you can neither prevent that problem nor can you coordinate the disease [management] well if you don't have coverage." (Families USA, July 12, 2005; Wonk Room, December 12, 2008)

Myth 9: Deregulating the healthcare industry will solve the health crisis. A recent *Washington Times* editorial suggested, "Let the marketplace answer both calls [of affordability and accessibility]. . . . The government cannot possibly do for Americans what the marketplace can." (*Washington Times*, December 15, 2008)

Reality: **The current marketplace is broken; it has failed to keep costs down and increase access to care.** Rather than competing on the value of care, insurance markets have "become dominated by a small number of large insurers" that don't use their market power to drive bargains with providers. The marketplace has contributed to skyrocketing premiums and huge cost shifts to families through higher deductibles and co-payments while largely excluding individuals with preexisting conditions from coverage. (Wonk Room, December 15, 2008)

Myth 10: Reform means forcing people to buy coverage they can't afford. Writing in the *Washington Times*, Michael Cannon, director of health policy studies at the Cato Institute, argues that "mandating that people purchase health insurance—on their own or through an employer—will increase its cost" and force "Americans to switch from their current health plan to a more expensive one, threatening their current source of care." (*Washington Times*, December 28, 2008)

Reality: **Extending coverage to all will provide Americans with insurance they can use.** Far from "forcing" Americans to buy more expensive coverage, progressives will ensure that Americans have access to a wide array of comprehensive insurance policies they can use if they become sick; a watered-down policy with high deductibles is no insurance at all. Americans who can't afford coverage will receive new tax credits to help make coverage more affordable and ensure that families don't spend more than a certain percentage of their income on health insurance premiums. (Progress Report, December 12, 2008)

Myth 11: Employer pay-or-play provisions will cost jobs. The *National Review* has argued that pay-or-play—a provision that requires large employers to either offer their employees coverage or pay into a fund that will help finance health insurance for their workers—would have "devastating" consequences "for the lowest paid workers." "These employers would therefore have no choice but to eliminate these jobs, lest they end up paying more for their workforce than it is worth to the firm." Conservatives also argue that "instead of bolstering private coverage, 'pay or play' would become the excuse for companies to drop their plans and push their employees into public insurance." (*National Review*, July 10, 2008)

Reality: **Employer mandates have not resulted in employers eliminating jobs.** Most large employers subject to a mandate already provide coverage to their workers. In fact, a recent Commonwealth Fund study of working-aged adults in Massachusetts—which has instituted an employer mandate—revealed that "employers have neither dropped coverage nor restricted eligibility for coverage in the state's first year of health reform." (Commonwealth Fund, October 28, 2008)

— part five —

A CALL TO ACTION

chapter fourteen

Know the Bottom Line

The bottom line on healthcare reform is that it is not worth doing if it is not done right.

It is important to distinguish between healthcare reform and insurance reform. There are pieces of the 2009 bill that don't cost any money.

The first is the issue of guaranteed insurance. As I explained previously, this means private insurance companies will not be able to drop patients once they become ill or attain a certain age. Private insurance companies will not be able to refuse any person who applies for insurance, regardless of preexisting conditions or age.

The second is community rating. This means private insurance companies will not be able to charge excessively more for people with significant illnesses or for the elderly.

These are essential parts of insurance reform because they make the insurance market fair and much more understandable to average people. As is the case in the Netherlands, France, and a number of other countries, the government can have a "regulator group," which would help in the private sector to smooth out the differences that can occur if one company, for whatever reason, were to acquire a disproportionate number of very ill or older patients.

Insurance reform is a good thing.

But that is not what Barack Obama promised the American people, it is not what Hillary Clinton promised the American people when she was a candidate, and it is not going to significantly change America's ability to control its costs or to make the insurance system work for the hundreds of thousands of healthcare professionals, hospitals, and other providers, let alone patients.

Real reform depends on one thing. That is patient choice. Real patient choice.

Americans must be free to have maximum choice in healthcare, and that includes a public option.

I have previously said that a Medicare-like program should be the public option. Medicare has its faults, as does every country's system, and as does the private sector. But Medicare is understandable. If you want this healthcare reform to pass, we first must make it understandable and reassure the American people that if they like what they have, they can keep it. Medicare is a well-respected, well-liked program. I would argue that if this bill is to pass with public support, the American public must understand that the choices they have all make sense and are also comfortable and familiar.

Today the American people have a choice of private insurers, sometimes employer-based and sometimes not. They understand those choices, even if they can't understand the policies, plans, or rules. They also understand Medicare. Almost all Americans are involved in some way with it. Their parents or grandparents may be beneficiaries, they may have another relative or a friend who is a beneficiary, or they may be on Medicare themselves. The vast majority of recipients are over sixty-five, but there are younger people with significant disabilities who could not get healthcare were it not for the Medicare system. This is particularly true of dialysis patients.

Medicare is familiar. By giving Americans a choice between a private sector plan and a Medicare-like program, we give them a choice between two knowns. They are more than capable of making this informed decision. To take away one of those choices is wrong.

We live in an age where we have just ended eight years of rule by those who would make our choices for us. They would tell us what is ideologically proper and then limit our choices to their lists. Public healthcare, other than the programs that existed when they got there, was not proper; therefore we had no choice to expand it. Deciding under what circumstances a woman would bear a child was not a debate they were willing to listen to, so they tried to restrict that choice and bar American women from making that choice for themselves. The core justice system could not be trusted to rule the way they wanted it to rule on the guilt or innocence of terrorists, so a separate system was invented so the core system would not have that choice. Americans in general, and Congress in particular, could not be trusted to assess the risks of Saddam Hussein and his dictatorship to U.S. security, so facts were withheld from Congress so they could not make an informed choice. Soldiers who chose to enlist to serve their country for a fixed period of time were suddenly denied the choice of leaving when the agreed-upon term of service was up. This was to serve the government's purpose.

Americans deserve real choice among options that may not be popular to either the left or the right. Those on the left who believe that everyone should be in a single-payer plan ought not be able to dictate to the American people who want a private insurance plan that they can't have one. American people deserve to make that choice. Those on the right who don't want an expansion of government and believe that the private sector can deliver everything necessary for a secure and fair society are entitled to choose private insurance. They are not, however, entitled to tell those who want to make a different choice that they can't.

Without this choice, there is no healthcare reform. Relying exclusively on private insurance for working-aged Americans has simply failed us. Our healthcare costs have risen over the last thirty years at two to three times the rate of inflation, a rate that is far higher than that of any other system in the world, where there is more government participation. The satisfaction rates with private sector American healthcare are lower than in any other industrialized democracy. In fact, every other industrialized democracy, including the most socialized system in the world, Great Britain's, has a choice. People can opt to get private insurance if they wish. If only conservatives could be as gracious in acknowledging our ability to make our own decisions as those on the left who would opt for more government involvement.

To deny the American people this choice is to deny healthcare reform at all. No doubt denying healthcare reform is high on the agenda of many in the American right wing. It is not, however, the sentiment that elected Barack Obama as president.

Subsidizing Americans to buy private health insurance without giving them the choice of a more rational and less expensive system is simply pouring money into a system that increases costs at twice the rate of inflation, serves preferentially those who don't need help, and offers no peace of mind to those at risk in difficult economic times.

In short, the healthcare reform bill is not worth passing unless the American people have the choice of signing up for a public option—a real public option. Some may craft a compromise that allows the public option to kick in at a later time. None of this is worth doing. Insurance reform is worth doing. If healthcare reform is not the desired outcome, this administration or the Democratic Party or the Congress as a whole should pass guaranteed issue and community rating and be done with it. These measures would not require any budget outlay, and our deficit situation would be much better in the short term. But if real healthcare reform as promised is to be delivered, the American people must have a real choice.

chapter fifteen

Meet Your Neighbors: You May Be One of Them

Most Americans eyes' glaze over when they have to think about healthcare reform. They don't know what reform will mean for them. It's expensive, it's complicated, and people can't visualize how their lives will change in a reformed healthcare system. That's why I've written below about how healthcare reform will affect seven fictional Americans in different income and employment situations. I want to explain in plain language what a reasonable, thoughtful healthcare reform bill will do for you.

Details of plans proposed in Congress may differ from the ideal plan I've built these cases upon, but if Congress does its job fairly and thoughtfully, this is what you should expect.

This is also what you deserve, and should fight for.

The low-wage worker: Sarah is a single mom whose husband walked out on her eight years ago. He rarely pays child support. She has two children in middle school and has supported them over the last eight years by working at various waitressing jobs, never making more than $28,000, including tips. She has no benefits and has never been able to even think about affording health insurance. She lives in Texas and her children are not eligible for SCHIP, the program that the federal government uses to help states give insurance to low-income children.

With real healthcare reform: Sarah's kids are eligible for SCHIP. She will get a generous subsidy to get private medical insurance or sign up for a public health insurance option (like Medicare).

No one knows what an exact plan would cost, but done right her payment could be about $100 per month.

What would happen in the current system? Sarah and her children would continue with no health insurance, which means that well-child and preventive care would not be done, and any serious health event—such as an accident for one of her children or herself—would lead to either bankruptcy or the family going on public assistance.

A part-time student with no financial support from parents: Jamal is a single twenty-five-year-old. He has been in and out of graduate school, getting by with part-time jobs in which he makes $15,000 a year, total. Both of his parents were killed in a car accident three years ago. After going through a difficult grieving period, Jamal vowed he would put his life back together and become a college professor. He has lived these last three years with no health insurance; its expense is unthinkable, despite the generous aid from the university for his part-time graduate student expenses. His parents, who had run their own small business, had borrowed against their life insurance policies in order to pay Jamal's undergraduate tuition, and the few assets left in their estate went to pay off business debt and to support his younger siblings.

With real healthcare reform: Under the Obama plan, Jamal would have a choice between signing up for a private insurance plan and joining the public insurance plan—likely to be the cheaper option. Because his income is so low, the vast majority of his premiums will be covered by the federal government. His out-of-pocket costs for public coverage might be about $50 to $100 per month.

What would happen in the current system? Jamal, like Sarah, is an automobile accident or an illness away from having his dreams, and his parents' dreams for him, destroyed.

Middle-income small business owners with children: John and Lena have a $70,000 household income and three small children, live just outside Cincinnati, and own their own retail business with three employees who make $10 an hour. They have a lot of employee turnover since they are unable to offer benefits. John bought health coverage for himself and his family with a $10,000-per-person deductible and a lifetime limit of $300,000 per family member. This type of policy might cost from $5,000 to $7,000 per year for a family of five.

With real healthcare reform: John, Lena, and their children are eligible for some government support, allowing them to choose between private health insurance and a public health insurance option. For about the same amount of money, they can get much better coverage with a modest deductible and co-payment, and lifetime limits that would run around $1 million per person if they chose private health insurance. (A $1 million lifetime exemption sounds like a lot, but it still does not protect a family should a major medical intervention such as heart or liver transplant be required. In the case of a Medicare-like plan, there are no lifetime limits.)

John and Lena would no longer have to worry about covering their employees. Like many small business employees, these workers would be able to enroll in either public or private insurance plans within the new health insurance pool. The government may subsidize their premiums on a sliding income scale.

What would happen in the current system? John and Lena would continue with very high-deductible insurance, one catastrophic illness away from losing their business and the jobs that go with it.

Professional parent of three, recently laid off: Manuel is a fifty-year-old recently laid off from his job as a computer programmer at a large bank. He was making $75,000 per year and now is able to string together some part-time consulting work that pays him $35,000 annually. He can't afford his COBRA payments—

which for him, his wife (who works part-time without benefits), and his high-school-aged children would come to $1,200 per month. The only way he could afford health insurance is to dip into his children's college funds, which he refuses to do. So, he and his family are currently uninsured.

With real healthcare reform: Manuel and his family are eligible to enroll in either a private health insurance plan or a public insurance option with government help. His cost to participate would likely be in the range of $300 to $400 per month, depending on his wife's income.

What would happen in the current system? Manuel and his wife continue to make the choice every month between educating their children after they leave high school and buying health insurance for their family. Manuel's job hunting is constrained because he needs to find a new employer who gives benefits.

Cancer survivor denied health insurance: Elizabeth is a single, forty-five-year-old self-employed woman who makes $150,000 per year. She is a breast cancer survivor. Her insurance company refused to renew her policy after paying out $200,000 worth of claims during her period of surgery and chemotherapy. She can afford health insurance, but no one will insure her because of her preexisting condition. In some ways Elizabeth is fortunate. Some insurance companies would have cut her off during her chemotherapy.

With real healthcare reform: Elizabeth can opt into a public health insurance plan that will cover her for the rest of her life without charging her any additional premiums due to her previous medical history. She will always be covered no matter where she lives, no matter what her occupation is—even if she becomes ill again and is disabled. She will not get a public subsidy unless her income drops far below where it is today. Her total premium will be no more than 20 percent higher than the premium for a healthy twenty-five-year-old man.

What would happen in the current system? Elizabeth would continue to live without health insurance. If she has a recurrence of her cancer, she would lose her business, and her life would likely be significantly shortened compared with those who can get adequate treatment because they are insured.

Employee of a major corporation: Glenn is a forty-three-year-old employee of a major high-tech firm with a full benefits package, 80 percent paid for by his company. He makes $60,000 a year. He has high blood pressure and a family history of heart disease.

With real healthcare reform: Glenn would be required to continue using his employer's insurance, unless the company chooses not to offer insurance as a benefit anymore. If the employer ends coverage, it would be required to make a contribution to a government fund. That contribution would be used to cover Glenn's health insurance cost. If Glenn loses his job, he can enroll in public or private health insurance and pay premiums based on his income.

What would happen in the current system? Good health insurance. If Glenn likes what he has, he can keep it. But if he loses his job or moves to another company, he is in trouble.

Prosperous executive wanting specialized family care: Jasmine is married and makes $200,000 per year at a small advertising agency. She has a diabetic son. Fortunately, her company has a group plan, which she currently uses. However, the company has announced that it is moving its headquarters across the country. Jasmine and her husband have decided it would be best not to make a move that would disrupt both his career and the carefully assembled medical support system for their son. While she has good insurance now, her husband works for himself. Unless Jasmine can find a job with a large company that offers group health insurance, it is likely that her next job would result in insurance that would cover only her and her husband, leaving her son vulnerable.

With real healthcare reform: Jasmine signs herself and her family up for a public health insurance option. While all her son's team accepts her coverage, she provides extra security by purchasing additional private insurance that covers nontraditional care.

What would happen in the current system? Jasmine will have difficulty getting private health insurance because of her son—unless she works in a company with group benefits.

chapter sixteen

What You Can Do for Your Neighbors, Your Country, and Yourself

The average American has more personal stake in the outcome of this legislative fight than in any other piece of legislation that will come before Congress for many, many years.

Until this recent election, which signified a generational change in American politics, the reaction of most citizens was to look at the congressional process with a sense of helplessness. The major actors in Washington appeared to be distant figures talking about complex matters. The media focused mostly on the political fighting and very little on substance. Consequently, many of the great battles over the past couple of decades have simply been condensed to sound bites and epithets hurled by opposing sides.

The generation that elected Barack Obama, however, has a different view of grassroots politics. They have learned to use the Internet—the greatest tool of democratization since the printing press was invented more than 500 years ago—to circumvent the traditional political process, form people-powered interest groups, and spread information electronically. Yet for those readers who are not part of this extraordinary new multicultural generation, which is so Internet-savvy, here are some things you can do.

First, go to the Web site StandwithDrDean.com. This is a site created by Democracy for America, a grassroots organization that sprang out of my presidential campaign more than five years ago. There are online petitions, organizing tools, and campaigns to contact your senators and congressmen to let them know how strongly you feel about Americans' right to choose whether they want a public health insurance option or to continue with their current health insurer.

Also, begin educating yourself about the legislative debate if you aren't already doing so. A number of leading bloggers such as Ezra Klein, Jonathan Cohn, ThinkProgress and its policy blog the Wonk Room, Talking Points Memo, the Huffington Post, and so many other progressive online reporting outfits do a fantastic job of keeping track of the day-to-day ups and downs of the health-care debate. Then start writing. Letters to the editors in your local paper matter; letters and e-mails to your congressmembers do, too.

Just as important as contacting your elected officials is contacting your fellow Americans. Door-knocking campaigns, such as the neighbor-to-neighbor approach that we used when I was chair of the Democratic National Committee, are an incredibly effective way of talking to people, building relationships, and communicating information.

Most Americans respond well to people they know. You should organize door-knocking teams to talk with people you know in your neighborhood or organize door-knocking teams so that one person has repeated interaction (dropping a flyer at the door is not enough) with the same person in each household until a relationship is established. Widening the circle using not just the Internet but also personal interaction gives this movement for real choice in our healthcare system much more impact.

People who are on television need to hear from you, too. Washington is an extraordinarily insular place. The culture in Washington is different from the culture in the rest of America. Everyone talks to one another in a relatively small and relatively closed circle. People who vote in Congress talk to a lot of media people, attorneys, lobbyists, and so on, who may not have a vote but who are part of the opinion-making crew in DC. They need to hear from you, too, because their opinions are listened to by those in Congress.

Contact major companies. It is no accident that the health insurance industry is taking on a much more conciliatory tone during this debate than it did during the healthcare debate during the Clinton years. They've heard from you. But don't be fooled. While their rhetoric may be conciliatory, their intention is to derail or manipulate this effort at healthcare reform so they can continue their march toward greater and greater earnings.

Contact other organizations that may be active in your community, particularly those that work at the grassroots level. Health Care for America Now (HCAN) is a Washington-based coalition that has national reach. MoveOn.org has been very active in support of a public plan. The Service Employees International Union and other labor unions have been active and supportive of a maximum range of healthcare choice. If you are a member of one of these organizations or know someone who is, find out what you can do to help.

Successful political campaigns never stop. America has seen one of the most successful campaigns ever run by the president. The campaign is not over. Electing a new president is only the beginning. We have to campaign every day for the next eight years to make sure this president has an agenda that we can support and that we fully support that agenda.

The purpose of electing a Democratic president was not simply to elect a Democratic president. The purpose of electing a Democratic president was to have in office a president who cares about ordinary people, and who is willing to fight hard for principles against the well-heeled forces in our nation's capital that resist change at every turn.

This is your fight. This is not a fight about what Barack Obama or Howard Dean or SEIU or MoveOn.org or Democracy for America want for all of us. As was the case in the Obama campaign, the battle is not won by the people who are running for office or running the campaign. Fights like this are won by ordinary people who decide that they care enough about something to fight for it. That is our challenge.

Index

About the Authors

Howard Dean—physician and former chairman of the Democratic National Committee (DNC)—served six terms as Governor of Vermont before running for the Democratic Party's presidential nomination in the 2004 election. A pioneer in the Netroots movement, Dean also founded Democracy for America (DFA), the grassroots organization that organizes community activists, trains campaign staff, and endorses progressive candidates. His experience as a practicing physician made him a career-long advocate of healthcare reform. While he was Vermont's governor, the state expanded its healthcare program to cover nearly every child under age 18—and also lowered its public debt, balanced its budget, and reduced taxes. In his four-year term as DNC chair, Dean originated and successfully implemented the party's 50-State Strategy, which focused on winning elections and organizing Democrats at every level in every region of the country, not just the states required to win presidential elections. A longtime champion of progressive politics and grassroots activism, he is chairman of the Progressive Book Club.

Igor Volsky is a healthcare researcher at the Center for American Progress. He blogs daily about healthcare reform at the Wonk Room (www.wonkroom.org). Igor studied history at Marist College and grew up in Russia, Israel, and New Jersey.

Faiz Shakir, currently the Research Director at the Center for American Progress, has been a researcher for the Democratic National Committee, a U.S. Senate legislative aide on veterans affairs, and a White House communications aide. He holds a B.A. in government from Harvard University and a J.D. from the Georgetown Law Center.